DELICIOUS WHOLE FOOD COOKBOOK

pil

Publications International, Ltd.

Some of the products listed in this publication may be in limited distribution.

Pictured on the front cover: Chicken with Quinoa Salad *(page 50)*.

Pictured on the back cover *(top to bottom)*: Chickpea Burgers *(page 52)*, Penne Pasta with Chunky Tomato Sauce and Spinach *(page 62)*, and Whole Wheat Pancakes *(page 5)*.

Photo on cover and on pages 51 and 115 © Shutterstock.com.

ISBN: 978-1-64558-746-0

Manufactured in China.

8 7 6 5 4 3 2 1

Microwave Cooking: Microwave ovens vary in wattage. Use the cooking times as guidelines and check for doneness before adding more time.

Let's get social!
⊙ @Publications_International
ⓕ @PublicationsInternational
www.pilbooks.com

TABLE OF
CONTENTS

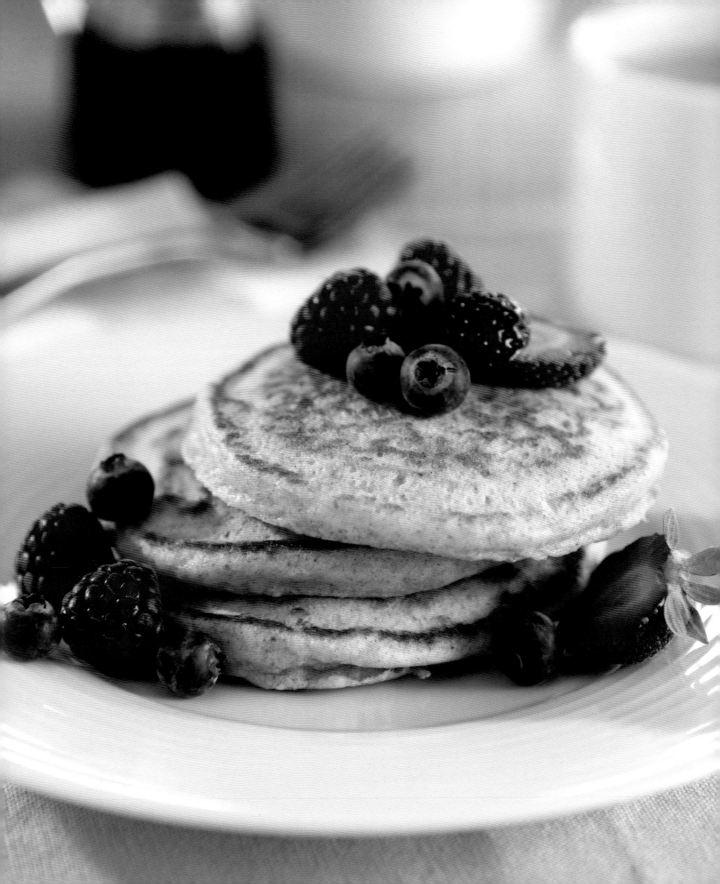

BOUNTIFUL BREAKFASTS

WHOLE WHEAT PANCAKES

¾ cup fat-free (skim) milk

2 eggs

¼ cup plain nonfat Greek yogurt

2 tablespoons vegetable oil

1 tablespoon honey

1 cup whole wheat flour

2 teaspoons baking powder

⅛ teaspoon salt

2 teaspoons butter

Fresh raspberries, blueberries and/or strawberries (optional)

Maple syrup or agave nectar (optional)

1 Whisk milk, eggs, yogurt, oil and honey in medium bowl until well blended. Add flour, baking powder and salt; whisk just until blended.

2 Heat large nonstick skillet over medium heat. Add 1 teaspoon butter; brush to evenly coat skillet. Drop batter by ¼ cupfuls into skillet. Cook 2 minutes or until tops of pancakes appear dull and bubbles form around edges. Turn and cook 1 to 2 minutes or until firm and bottoms are browned, adding remaining 1 teaspoon butter as needed.

3 Top with berries and maple syrup, if desired.

Tip

To keep pancakes warm while remaining batches are cooking, preheat oven to 200°F and place a wire cooling rack directly on oven rack. Transfer pancakes to wire rack as they finish cooking. The pancakes will stay warm without getting soggy.

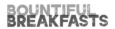

FRITTATA RUSTICA

4 ounces cremini mushrooms, stems trimmed, cut into thirds

1 tablespoon olive oil, divided

½ teaspoon plus ⅛ teaspoon salt, divided

½ cup chopped onion

1 cup packed chopped stemmed lacinato kale

½ cup halved grape tomatoes

4 eggs

½ teaspoon Italian seasoning

Black pepper

⅓ cup shredded mozzarella cheese

1 tablespoon shredded Parmesan cheese

Chopped fresh parsley (optional)

1 Preheat oven to 400°F. Spread mushrooms on small baking sheet; drizzle with 1 teaspoon oil and sprinkle with ⅛ teaspoon salt. Roast 15 to 20 minutes or until well browned and tender.

2 Heat remaining 2 teaspoons oil in small nonstick ovenproof skillet over medium heat. Add onion; cook and stir 5 minutes or until soft. Add kale and ¼ teaspoon salt; cook and stir 10 minutes or until kale is tender. Add tomatoes; cook and stir 3 minutes or until tomatoes are soft. Stir in mushrooms.

3 Preheat broiler. Whisk eggs, remaining ¼ teaspoon salt, Italian seasoning and pepper in small bowl until well blended.

4 Pour egg mixture over vegetables in skillet; stir gently to mix. Cook 3 minutes or until eggs are set around edge, lifting edge to allow uncooked portion to flow underneath. Sprinkle with mozzarella and Parmesan cheese.

5 Broil 3 minutes or until eggs are set and cheese is browned. Garnish with parsley.

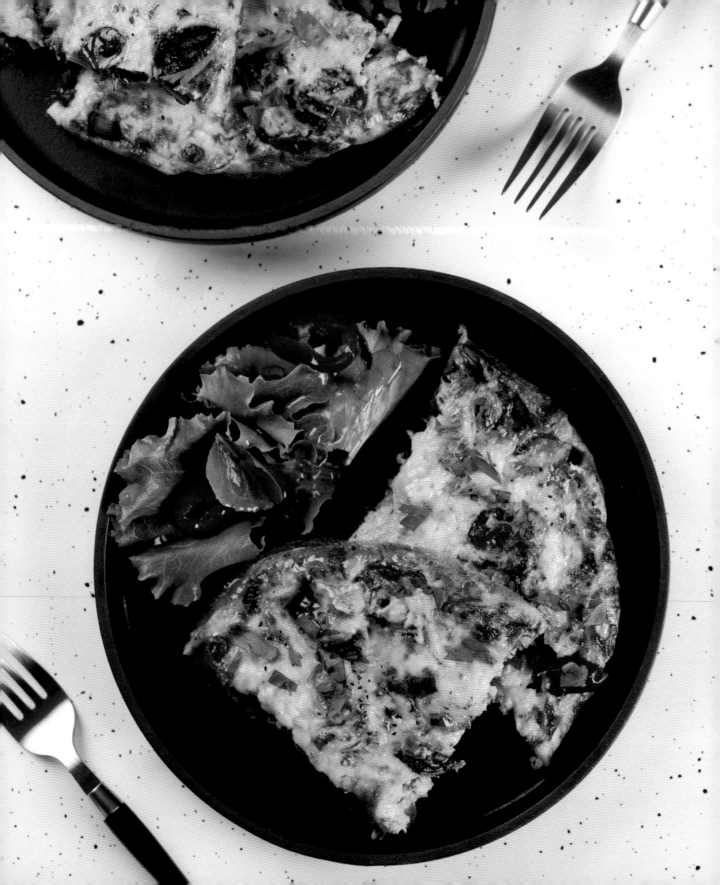

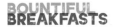

DATE-NUT GRANOLA

2 cups old-fashioned oats

2 cups barley flakes

1 cup sliced almonds

⅓ cup vegetable oil

⅓ cup honey

1 teaspoon vanilla

1 cup chopped dates

1 Preheat oven to 350°F. Spray 13×9-inch baking pan with nonstick cooking spray.

2 Combine oats, barley flakes and almonds in large bowl. Combine oil, honey and vanilla in small bowl; mix well. Pour syrup mixture over oat mixture; stir until well blended. Spread in prepared pan.

3 Bake about 25 minutes or until toasted, stirring frequently after 10 minutes. Stir in dates while granola is still hot. Cool. Store tightly covered.

Vegan Variation

Replace honey with agave syrup.

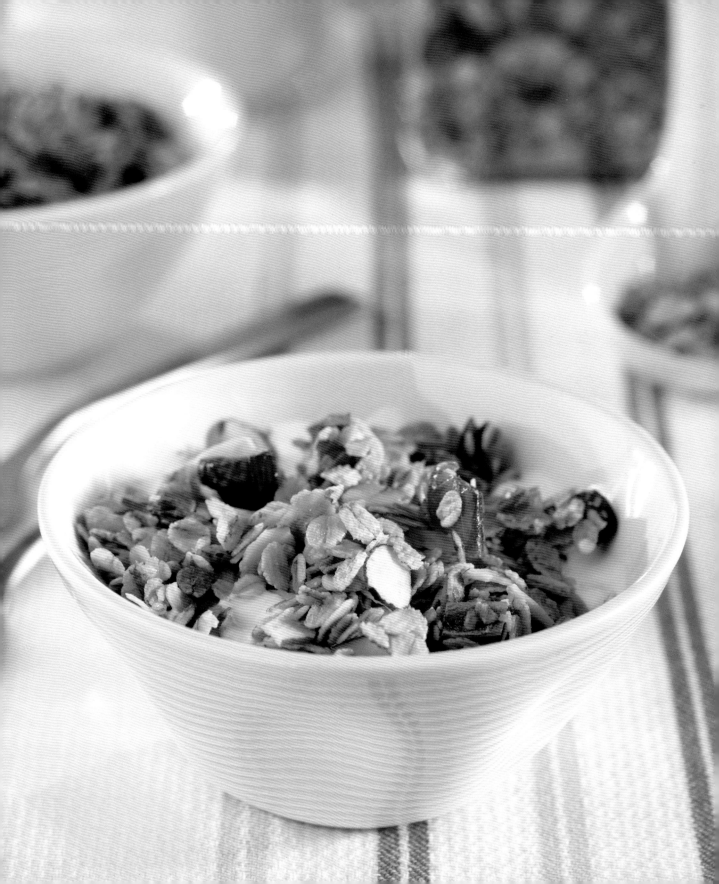

CRANBERRY
BUTTERMILK PANCAKES

MAKES ABOUT 6 SERVINGS

1 cup all-purpose flour

1 cup whole wheat flour

2 teaspoons baking powder

1 teaspoon baking soda

½ teaspoon ground cinnamon

¼ teaspoon ground nutmeg

⅔ cup whole berry cranberry
   sauce, divided

2 eggs

2 tablespoons vegetable oil

1½ cups low-fat buttermilk

   Maple syrup (optional)

1 Combine all-purpose flour, whole wheat flour, baking powder, baking soda, cinnamon and nutmeg in small bowl; mix well. Whisk cranberry sauce, eggs and oil in large bowl until well blended. Gradually stir in flour mixture until combined. Stir in buttermilk until smooth and well blended.

2 Heat large nonstick skillet or griddle over medium heat. Pour ¼ cupfuls of batter 2 inches apart onto griddle. Cook 3 minutes or until lightly browned and edges begin to bubble. Turn over; cook 3 minutes or until lightly browned. Repeat with remaining batter. Serve with maple syrup, if desired.

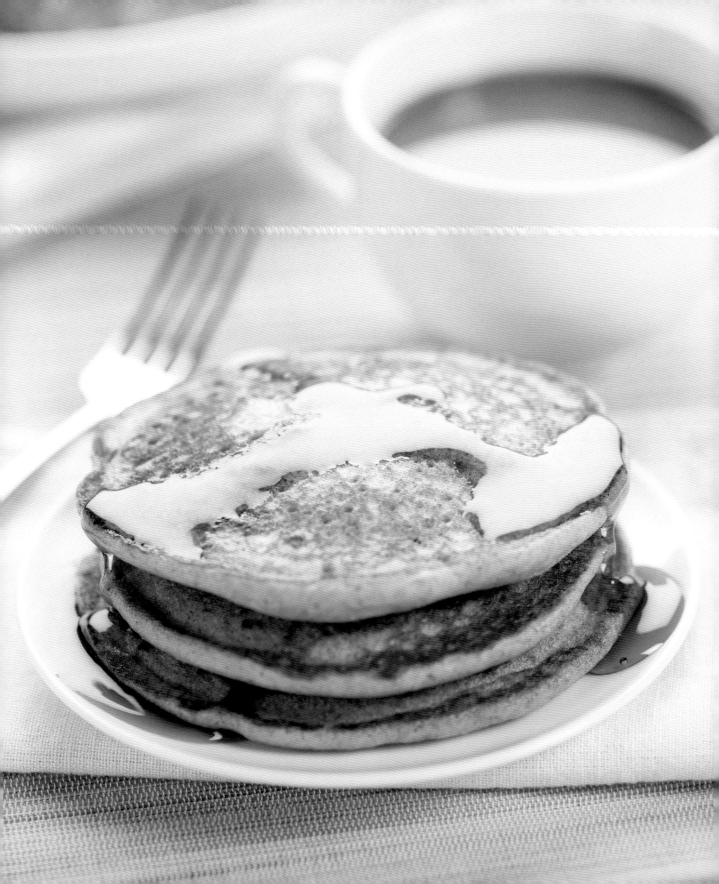

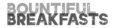

QUINOA & OAT MUESLI

1 cup uncooked quinoa

3 cups old-fashioned rolled oats

¼ cup unsweetened flaked coconut

¾ cup coarsely chopped almonds

½ teaspoon ground cinnamon

½ cup toasted wheat germ

¼ cup ground flaxseed

1¼ cups dried or freeze-dried fruit

1 Preheat oven to 350°F. Spread quinoa in single layer on baking sheet. Bake 8 to 10 minutes or until toasted and golden brown, stirring frequently. (Quinoa will make a slight popping sound when almost done.) Remove to large bowl; cool completely.

2 Combine oats, coconut, almonds and cinnamon on same baking sheet; mix well. Spread in even layer. Bake 15 minutes or until mixture is toasted and fragrant but not burnt. Let cool completely.

3 Add oat mixture to cooled quinoa in large bowl. Stir in wheat germ, flaxseed and dried fruit.

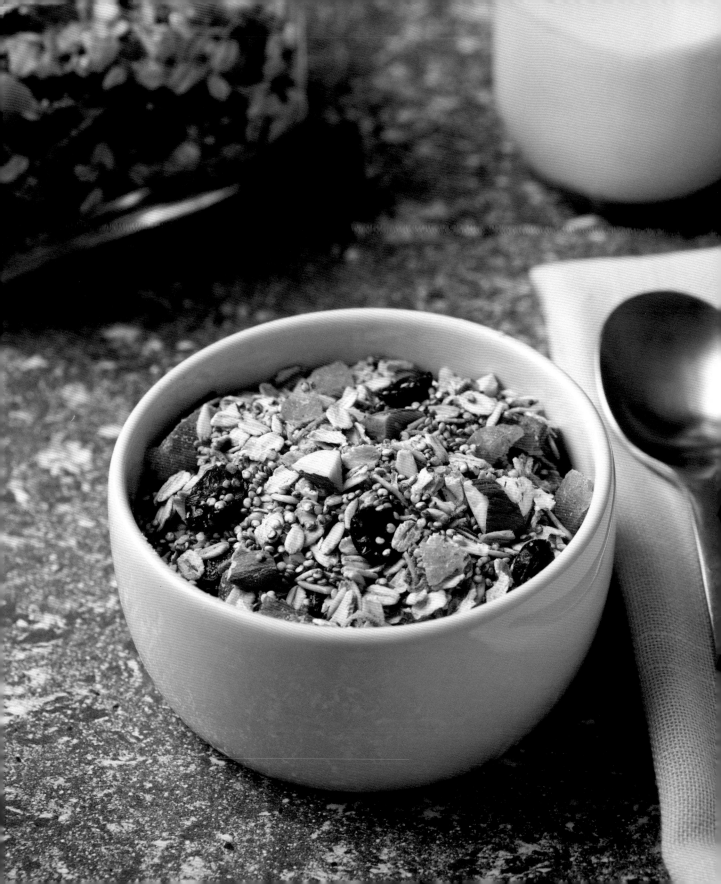

VANILLA MULTIGRAIN WAFFLES

MAKES 4 WAFFLES

1 cup low-fat buttermilk

¼ cup steel-cut oats

⅓ cup all-purpose flour

⅓ cup whole wheat flour

1 teaspoon baking powder

½ teaspoon baking soda

¼ teaspoon salt

1 egg

2 tablespoons packed brown sugar

1 tablespoon vegetable oil

1 teaspoon vanilla

Maple syrup (optional)

1 Combine buttermilk and oats in large bowl; let stand 10 minutes. Spray waffle maker with nonstick cooking spray; preheat according to manufacturer's directions.

2 Combine all-purpose flour, whole wheat flour, baking powder, baking soda and salt in medium bowl; mix well.

3 Whisk egg, brown sugar, oil and vanilla in small bowl until smooth and well blended. Stir into oat mixture. Add flour mixture; stir until smooth and well blended.

4 Pour ⅔ cup batter into waffle maker; cook about 5 minutes or until steam stops escaping from around edges and waffle is golden brown. Repeat with remaining batter. Serve with maple syrup, if desired.

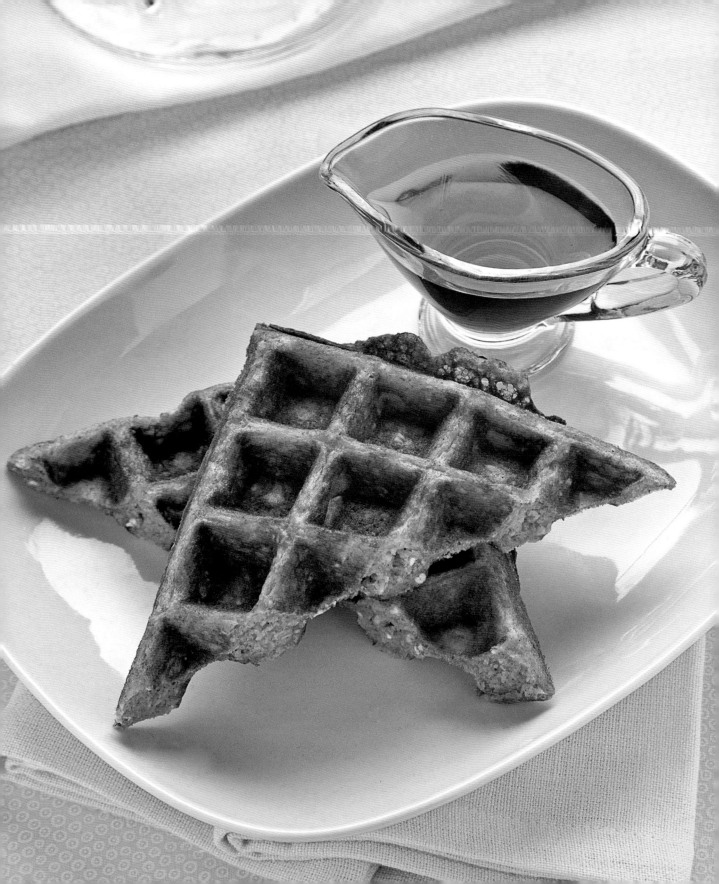

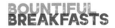

APPLE-CINNAMON BREAKFAST RISOTTO

MAKES 6 SERVINGS

¼ cup (½ stick) butter

4 medium Granny Smith apples, peeled and diced (about 1½ pounds)

1½ teaspoons ground cinnamon

¼ teaspoon salt

¼ teaspoon ground allspice

1½ cups uncooked arborio rice

½ cup packed dark brown sugar

4 cups unfiltered apple juice,* at room temperature

1 teaspoon vanilla

Milk (optional)

Sliced almonds and dried cranberries (optional)

If unfiltered apple juice is unavailable, use any apple juice.

Slow Cooker Directions

1 Melt butter in large skillet over medium-high heat. Add apples, cinnamon, salt and allspice; cook and stir 3 to 5 minutes or until apples begin to soften.

2 Combine apple mixture and rice in slow cooker; stir to coat. Sprinkle evenly with brown sugar. Add apple juice and vanilla. Cover; cook on HIGH 1½ to 2 hours or until all liquid is absorbed.

3 Spoon risotto into 6 serving bowls. Serve with milk and garnish with almonds and cranberries, if desired.

Note

Arborio rice, an Italian-grown short grain rice, has a delicious nutty taste. It is traditionally used for risotto dishes because its high starch content produces a creamy texture. The large, plump grain is nearly flavorless, so it can be used for sweet and savory dishes for someone on a gluten-free diet.

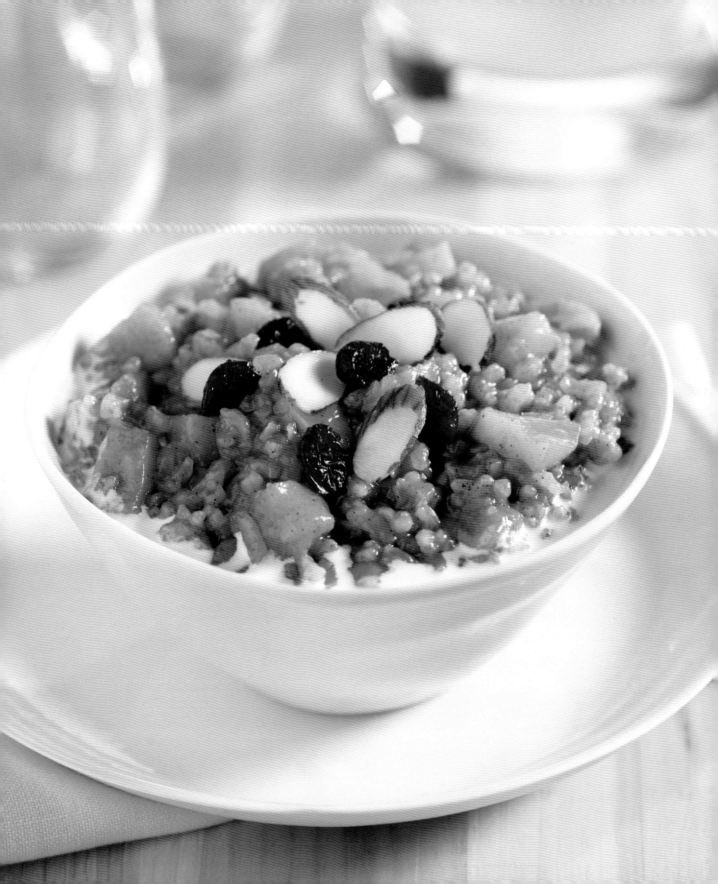

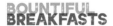
BLUEBERRY AND BRAN GRANOLA

MAKES 8 SERVINGS

½ cup dried blueberries

½ cup finely chopped dried apples

½ cup chopped walnuts

½ teaspoon ground cinnamon

½ teaspoon vanilla

1 tablespoon honey

2½ cups bran flakes

1 Preheat oven to 300°F. Coat large rimmed baking pan or jelly roll pan with nonstick cooking spray. Stir together blueberries, apples, walnuts, cinnamon, vanilla and honey in large bowl; mix well. Fold in bran flakes.

2 Spread mixture in prepared pan. Bake about 10 minutes, stirring halfway through baking time, or until mixture is browned and aromatic. Cool to room temperature before serving. Store in tightly covered container.

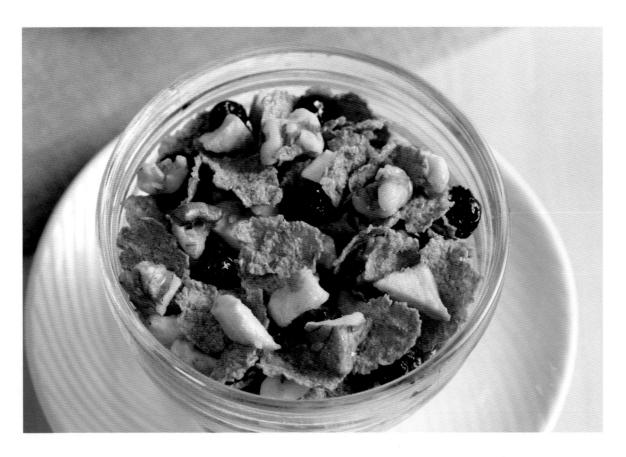

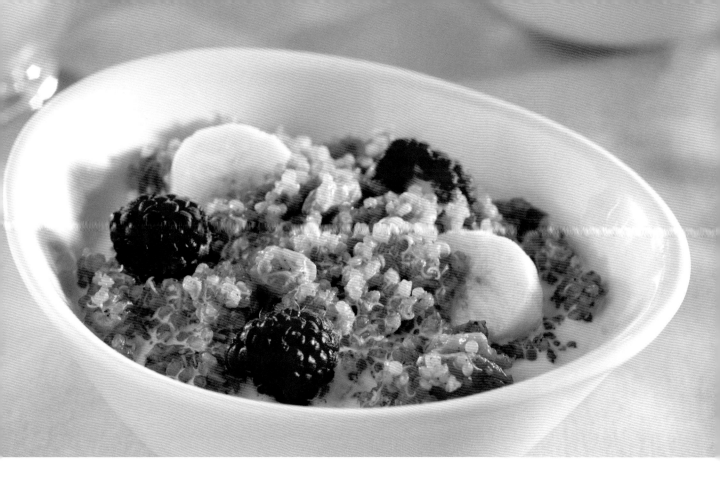

BREAKFAST QUINOA

½ cup uncooked quinoa

1 cup water

1 tablespoon packed brown sugar

2 teaspoons maple syrup

½ teaspoon ground cinnamon

½ teaspoon salt

¼ cup golden raisins (optional)

Reduced-fat (2%) milk (optional)

¼ cup fresh raspberries

½ banana, sliced

1 Place quinoa in fine-mesh strainer; rinse well under cold running water. Transfer to small saucepan.

2 Stir in 1 cup water, brown sugar, maple syrup, cinnamon and salt; bring to a boil over high heat. Reduce heat to low; cover and simmer 10 to 15 minutes or until quinoa is tender and water is absorbed. Add raisins, if desired, during last 5 minutes of cooking. Serve with milk, if desired; top with raspberries and bananas.

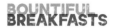

FRUITY WHOLE GRAIN CEREAL

MAKES 4 TO 6 SERVINGS

- 2 cups water
- ¼ cup uncooked instant oats
- ¼ cup uncooked quick-cooking barley
- ¼ cup uncooked instant whole grain brown rice
- ¼ teaspoon salt
- ½ cup milk
- ⅓ cup golden raisins
- ¼ cup finely chopped dried dates
- ¼ cup chopped dried plums
- 2 tablespoons packed brown sugar
- ½ teaspoon ground cinnamon

1 Combine water, oats, barley, rice and salt in large saucepan; bring to a boil over high heat. Reduce heat to low; cover and simmer 8 minutes or until rice and barley are tender but still slightly firm.

2 Stir in milk, raisins, dates, plums, brown sugar and cinnamon; mix well. Cover and simmer 3 to 5 minutes or until cereal is creamy, stirring occasionally. Serve hot. Refrigerate any leftover cereal in airtight container.

Tip

To reheat cereal, place one serving in microwavable bowl. Microwave on HIGH 30 seconds; stir. Add water or milk to reach desired consistency. Microwave just until hot.

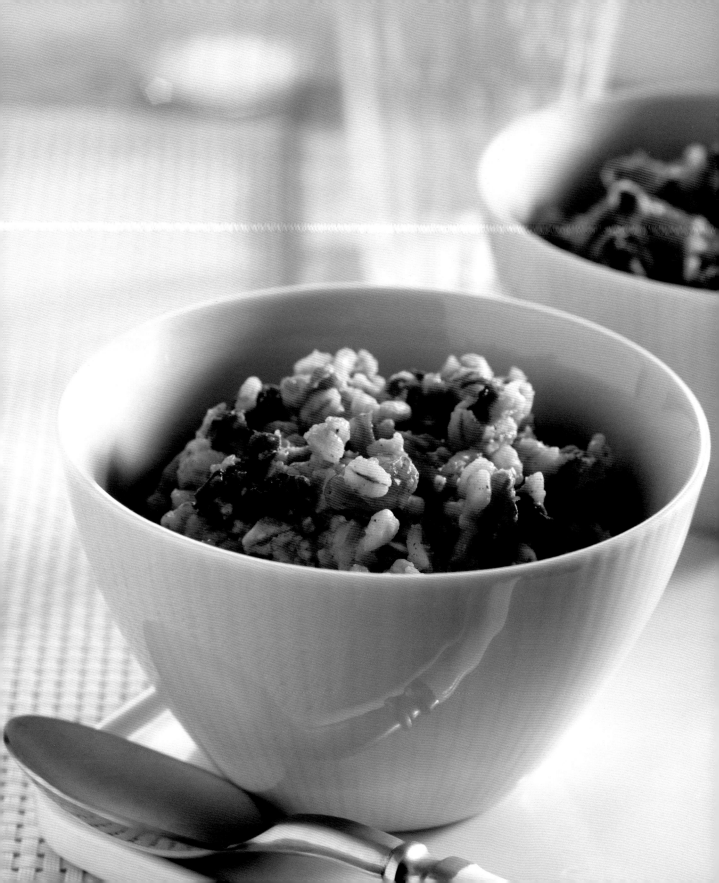

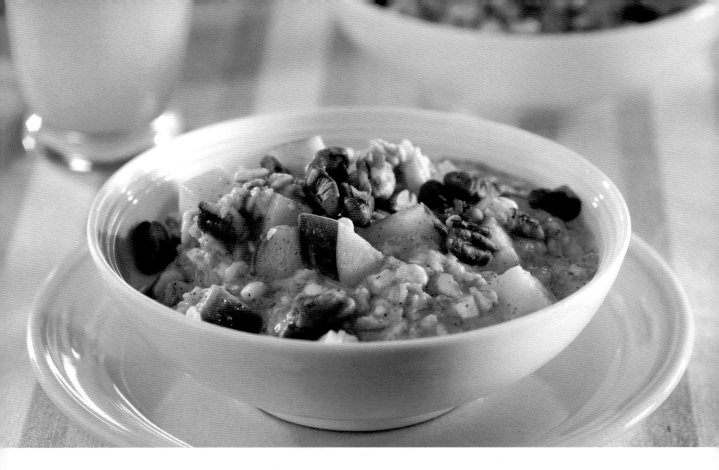

OATMEAL WITH APPLES AND COTTAGE CHEESE

MAKES 2 SERVINGS

⅔ cup water

¼ teaspoon salt

½ cup old-fashioned oats

½ cup diced apple

2 tablespoons packed brown sugar, granulated sugar or raw sugar

1 teaspoon vanilla

¾ teaspoon ground cinnamon

½ cup cottage cheese

¼ cup half-and-half

2 tablespoons chopped pecans or almonds

1 Bring water and salt to a boil in small saucepan over high heat. Stir in oats, apple, sugar, vanilla and cinnamon. Reduce heat to medium-low; cook and stir 3 to 5 minutes or until oats are tender and creamy.

2 Stir in cottage cheese and half-and-half; spoon into serving bowls. Top with nuts.

SUPER OATMEAL

2 cups water

2¾ cups old-fashioned oats

½ cup finely diced dried figs

½ cup sliced almonds, toasted*

⅓ cup packed dark brown sugar

¼ cup flaxseed

½ teaspoon salt

½ teaspoon ground cinnamon

2 cups reduced-fat (2%) milk, plus additional for serving

To toast almonds, spread in single layer in heavy skillet. Cook over medium heat 2 to 3 minutes or until lightly browned, stirring frequently.

1 Bring water to a boil in large saucepan over high heat. Stir in oats, figs, almonds, brown sugar, flaxseed, salt and cinnamon. Add 2 cups milk; mix well.

2 Reduce heat to medium. Cook and stir 5 to 7 minutes or until oatmeal is thick and creamy. Spoon into individual bowls. Serve with additional milk, if desired.

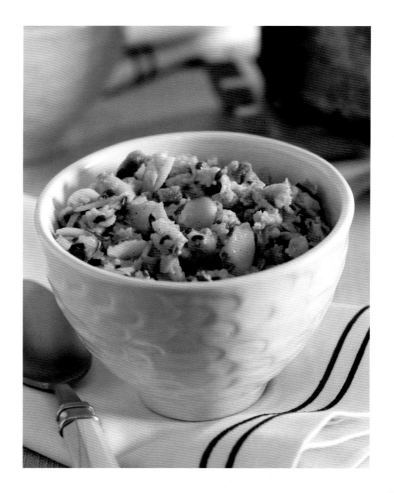

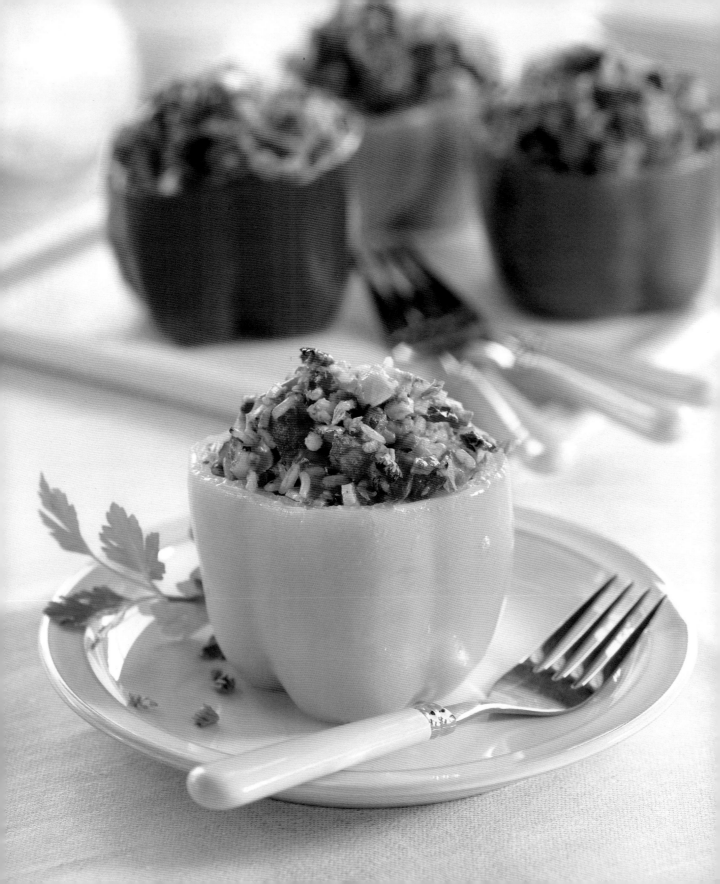

ENTICING ENTRÉES

PEPPERS STUFFED WITH YELLOW SQUASH AND RICE

MAKES 4 SERVINGS

½ cup long-grain brown rice (makes 1¾ cups cooked)

5 large green, red or yellow bell peppers, divided

2 teaspoons olive oil

2 medium yellow squash (1 pound), chopped

1 small onion, diced

2 cloves garlic, minced

1 large tomato, chopped

½ cup tomato sauce

3 tablespoons chopped fresh basil or parsley

¼ teaspoon salt

⅛ teaspoon black pepper

½ cup Parmesan cheese

1 Cook rice according to package directions.

2 Preheat oven to 400°F. Bring large pot of water to a boil. Slice off tops from 4 bell peppers; scrape out centers to remove seeds and membranes. Place bell peppers into boiling water; cook 4 minutes to soften slightly. Use slotted spoon to remove from boiling water; set aside.

3 Chop remaining bell pepper. Heat oil in large nonstick skillet over medium-high heat. Add chopped bell pepper, squash and onion; cook, stirring frequently, until softened, 5 minutes. Add garlic; cook and stir 1 minute. Add cooked rice, tomato and tomato sauce; cook until heated through. Stir in parsley, salt, black pepper and Parmesan cheese.

4 Spray 13×9-inch baking dish with nonstick cooking spray. Fill each bell pepper with about ½ cup rice mixture. Arrange stuffed peppers in single layer in baking dish. Bake, uncovered, 25 to 30 minutes or until bell peppers are heated through.

WHOLE WHEAT PENNE PASTA WITH SUMMER VEGETABLES

MAKES 4 SERVINGS

6 ounces uncooked whole wheat penne pasta (about 2 cups)

2 teaspoons olive oil

2 cloves garlic, minced

1½ cups chopped fresh broccoli

1 medium zucchini, chopped (about 1¼ cups)

½ medium yellow bell pepper, chopped (about ¾ cup)

8 ounces (about 1½ cups) cherry or grape tomatoes, halved

3 ounces (about 1 cup) mushrooms, sliced

½ teaspoon dried oregano

¾ cup crumbled feta cheese

1 Cook pasta according to package directions, omitting any salt or fat. Drain and keep warm.

2 Heat oil in large nonstick skillet over medium-high heat. Add garlic, broccoli, zucchini and bell pepper. Cook and stir about 2 minutes or until vegetables just begin to soften.

3 Add tomatoes, mushrooms and oregano; mix well. Reduce heat to medium and cook and stir about 8 minutes or until vegetables are tender and tomatoes release their juices.

4 Toss vegetables with pasta. Top with feta cheese.

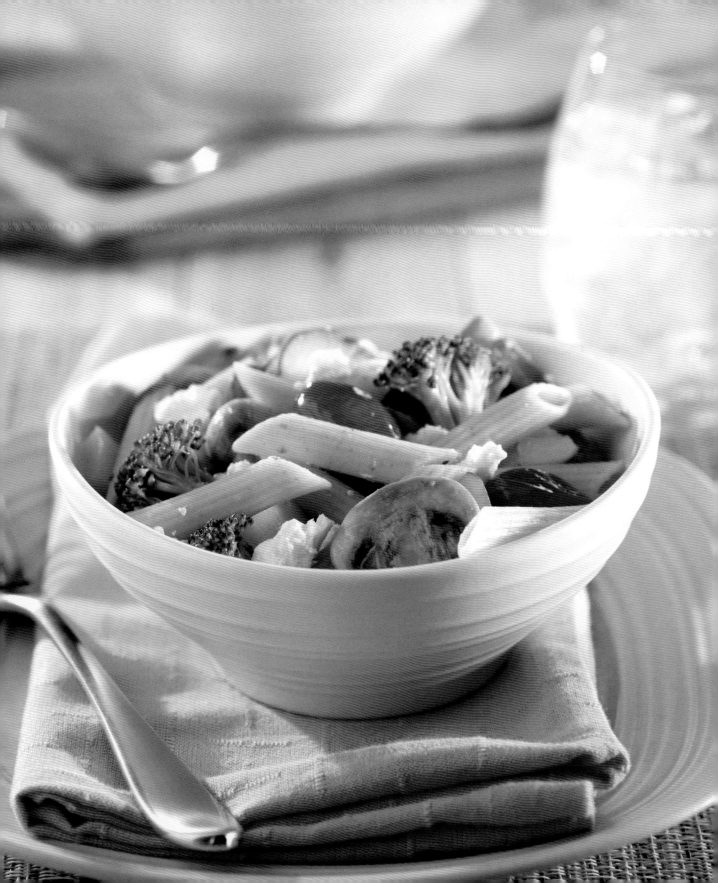

ISLAND
FISH TACOS

Coleslaw

1 medium jicama (about
   12 ounces), peeled and
   shredded

2 cups packaged coleslaw mix

3 tablespoons finely chopped
   fresh cilantro

¼ cup lime juice

¼ cup vegetable oil

3 tablespoons white vinegar

2 tablespoons mayonnaise

1 tablespoon honey

1 teaspoon salt

Salsa

2 medium fresh tomatoes,
   diced (about 2 cups)

½ cup finely chopped red
   onion

¼ cup finely chopped fresh
   cilantro

2 tablespoons lime juice

2 tablespoons minced
   jalapeño pepper*

1 teaspoon salt

*Jalapeño peppers can sting and
irritate the skin, so wear rubber
gloves when handling peppers and
do not touch your eyes.*

Tacos

1 to 1¼ pounds white fish such as
   tilapia or mahi mahi, cut into
   3×1½-inch pieces

Salt and black pepper

2 tablespoons vegetable oil

12 (6-inch) taco-size tortillas, heated

Prepared guacamole (optional)

1 For coleslaw, combine jicama, coleslaw mix and
  3 tablespoons cilantro in medium bowl. Whisk
  ¼ cup lime juice, ¼ cup oil, vinegar, mayonnaise,
  honey and 1 teaspoon salt in small bowl until well
  blended. Pour over vegetable mixture; stir to coat.
  Let stand at least 15 minutes for flavors to blend.

2 For salsa, place tomatoes in fine-mesh strainer; set
  in bowl or sink to drain 15 minutes. Remove to
  another medium bowl. Stir in onion, ¼ cup cilantro,
  2 tablespoons lime juice, jalapeño pepper and
  1 teaspoon salt; mix well.

3 For tacos, season both sides of fish with salt and
  black pepper. Heat 1 tablespoon oil in large nonstick
  skillet over medium-high heat. Add half of fish;
  cook 2 minutes per side or until fish is opaque and
  begins to flake when tested with fork. Repeat with
  remaining oil and fish.

4 Break fish into bite-size pieces; serve in tortillas with
  coleslaw, salsa and guacamole, if desired.

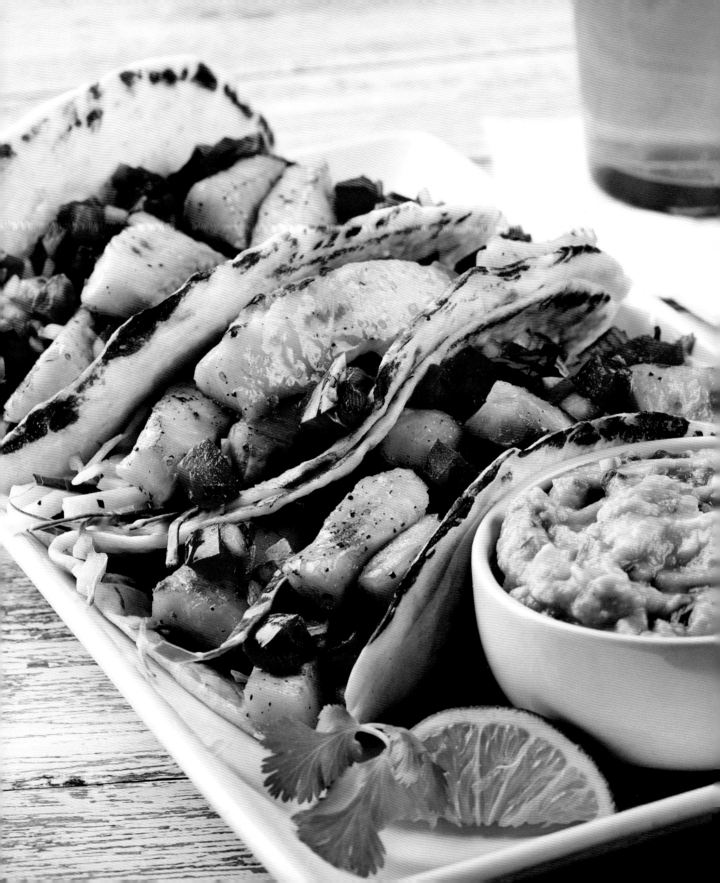

RICE NOODLES WITH BROCCOLI AND TOFU

MAKES 4 TO 6 SERVINGS

1 package (14 ounces) firm or extra firm tofu

1 package (8 to 10 ounces) wide rice noodles

2 tablespoons peanut oil

3 medium shallots, sliced

6 cloves garlic, minced

1 jalapeño pepper,* minced

2 teaspoons minced fresh ginger

3 cups broccoli florets

3 tablespoons regular soy sauce

1 tablespoon sweet soy sauce (kecap manis)**

1 to 2 tablespoons fish sauce

Fresh basil leaves (optional)

Jalapeño peppers can sting and irritate the skin, so wear rubber gloves when handling peppers and do not touch your eyes.

**If sweet soy sauce is not available, substitute 1 tablespoon soy sauce plus 1 tablespoon packed brown sugar.*

1 Cut tofu crosswise into 2 pieces. Place tofu on cutting board between layers of paper towels; place weighted saucepan or baking dish on top of tofu. Let stand 30 minutes to drain. Place rice noodles in large bowl; cover with boiling water. Soak 30 minutes or until soft.

2 Cut tofu into bite-size squares and blot dry. Heat oil in large skillet or wok over medium-high heat. Add tofu to skillet; stir-fry about 5 minutes or until tofu is lightly browned on all sides. Remove from skillet.

3 Add shallots, garlic, jalapeño pepper and ginger to skillet. Cook 2 to 3 minutes. Add broccoli; cook 1 minute. Cover and cook 3 minutes or until broccoli is crisp-tender.

4 Drain noodles. Add to skillet; stir to combine. Return tofu to skillet; add soy sauces and fish sauce. Cook 8 minutes or until noodles are coated and flavors are blended. Garnish with basil.

NOTE

To make this dish vegetarian, look for vegetarian fish sauce or substitute additional soy sauce or fresh lime juice.

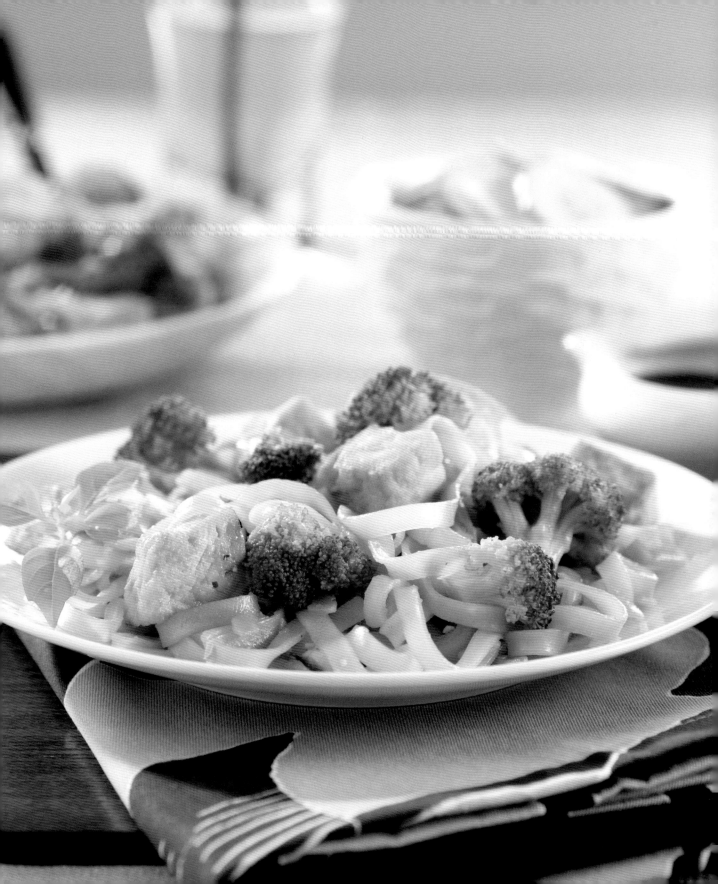

WHOLE WHEAT FLATBREAD WITH HERBED RICOTTA, PEACHES AND ARUGULA

MAKES 4 SERVINGS

½ cup ricotta cheese

2 tablespoons finely chopped fresh basil

½ teaspoon coarse salt

⅛ teaspoon black pepper

2 whole wheat naan breads

1 ripe peach, cut into 12 slices

½ cup arugula

½ teaspoon lemon juice

1 teaspoon extra virgin olive oil

2 teaspoons balsamic vinegar

Flaky sea salt, for sprinkling

1 Preheat oven to 400°F. Line baking sheet with parchment paper.

2 Combine ricotta, basil, coarse salt and pepper in small bowl; mix well. Spread mixture evenly over naan; top with peach slices.

3 Bake 12 minutes or until bottom of naan is crisp.

4 Combine arugula, lemon juice and oil in medium bowl; toss gently. Top baked flatbreads with arugula mixture; drizzle with vinegar and sprinkle with sea salt. Cut each flatbread into quarters.

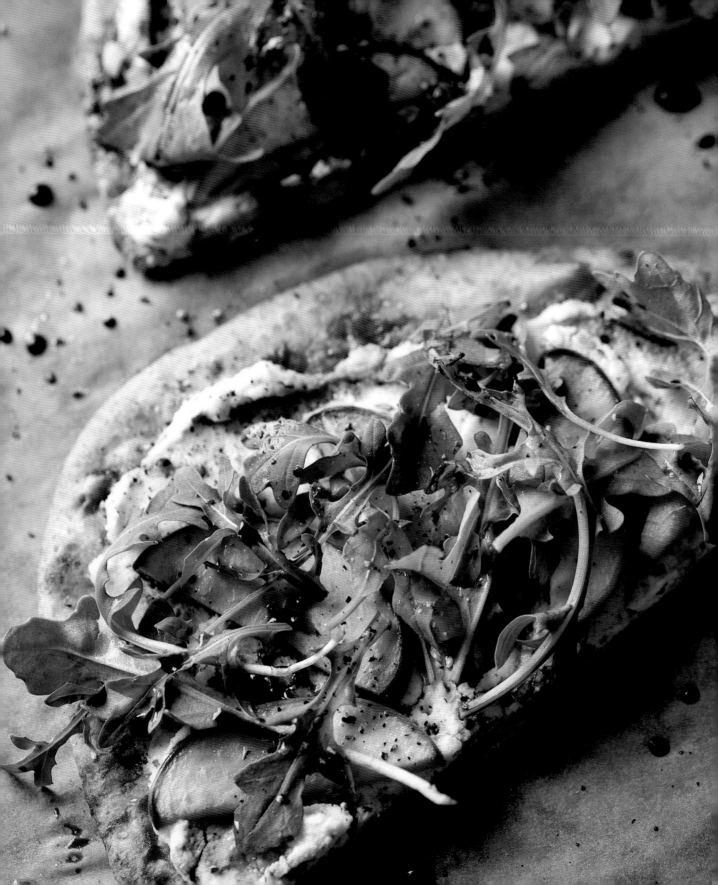

STEAK FAJITAS

¼ cup lime juice

¼ cup soy sauce

4 tablespoons vegetable oil, divided

2 tablespoons honey

2 tablespoons Worcestershire sauce

2 cloves garlic, minced

½ teaspoon ground red pepper

1 pound flank steak, skirt steak or top sirloin

1 medium yellow onion, halved and cut into ¼-inch slices

1 green bell pepper, cut into ¼-inch strips

1 red bell pepper, cut into ¼-inch strips

Flour tortillas, warmed

Lime wedges (optional)

Optional toppings: pico de gallo, guacamole, sour cream, shredded lettuce and shredded Cheddar-Jack cheese

1 Combine lime juice, soy sauce, 2 tablespoons oil, honey, Worcestershire sauce, garlic and ground red pepper in medium bowl; mix well. Remove ¼ cup marinade to large bowl. Place steak in large resealable food storage bag. Pour remaining marinade over steak; seal bag and turn to coat. Marinate in refrigerator at least 2 hours or overnight. Add onion and bell peppers to bowl with ¼ cup marinade; toss to coat. Cover and refrigerate until ready to use.

2 Remove steak from marinade; discard marinade and pat steak dry with paper towels. Heat 1 tablespoon oil in large skillet (preferably cast iron) over medium-high heat. Cook steak 4 minutes per side for medium rare or to desired doneness. Remove to large cutting board; tent with foil and let stand 10 minutes.

3 Meanwhile, heat remaining 1 tablespoon oil in same skillet over medium-high heat. Add vegetable mixture; cook 8 minutes or until vegetables are crisp-tender and beginning to brown in spots, stirring occasionally. (Cook in two batches if necessary; do not crowd vegetables in skillet.)

4 Cut steak into thin slices across the grain. Serve with vegetables, tortillas, lime wedges and desired toppings.

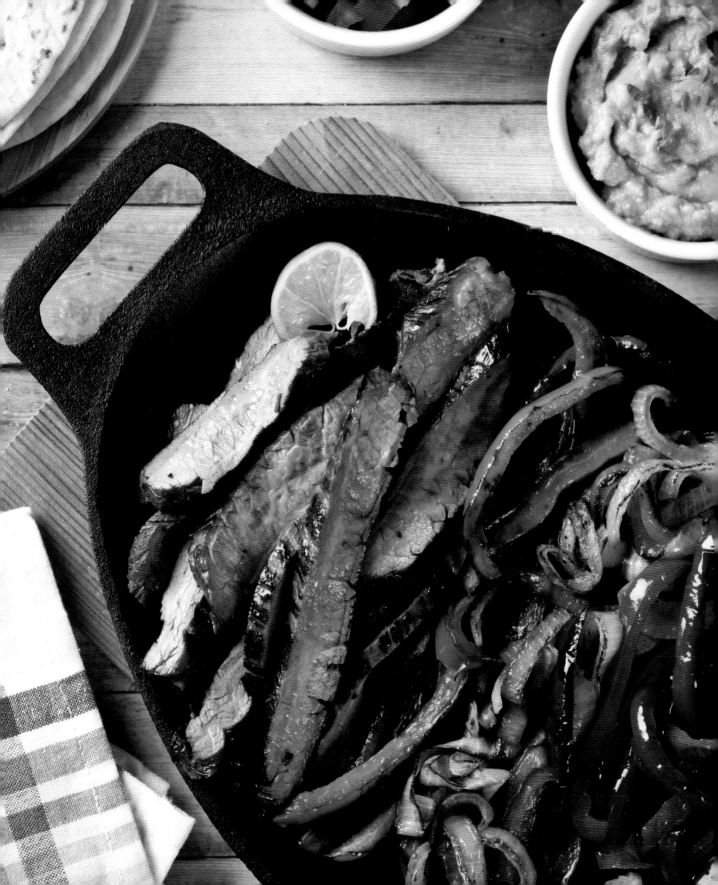

KALE, MUSHROOM AND CARAMELIZED ONION PIZZA

MAKES 4 SERVINGS

1 package (about 14 ounces) refrigerated pizza dough

1 tablespoon olive oil

1 cup small yellow onion, chopped

1 package (8 ounces) sliced mushrooms

3 cloves garlic, minced

4 cups packed coarsely chopped kale

¼ teaspoon red pepper flakes

½ cup pizza sauce

¾ cup (3 ounces) finely shredded part-skim mozzarella cheese

1 Preheat oven to 425°F. Spray 15×10-inch jelly-roll pan with nonstick cooking spray. Unroll pizza dough on prepared pan. Press dough evenly into pan and ½ inch up sides. Prick dough all over with fork. Bake 7 to 10 minutes or until lightly browned.

2 Heat oil in large nonstick skillet over medium heat. Add onion; cook and stir 8 minutes or until golden brown. Add mushrooms and garlic; cook and stir 4 minutes. Add kale and red pepper flakes; cover and cook 2 minutes to wilt kale. Uncover; cook and stir 3 to 4 minutes or until vegetables are tender.

3 Spread pizza sauce over crust. Spread kale mixture evenly over sauce; top with cheese. Bake 10 minutes or until crust is golden brown.

Note

Kale has tough stems that should be removed before cooking. To trim away tough stems, make a "V-shaped" cut where the stem joins the leaf. Stack the leaves and cut them into pieces.

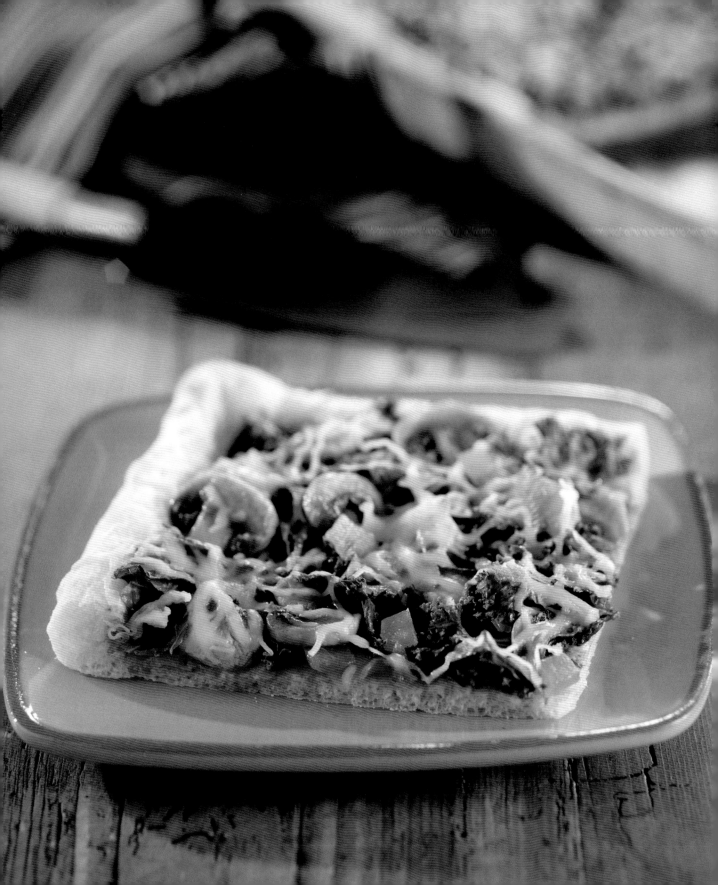

CILANTRO PEANUT PESTO ON SOBA

MAKES 4 TO 6 SERVINGS

1 cup packed fresh basil leaves

½ cup packed fresh cilantro leaves

¾ cup dry roasted peanuts, divided

1 jalapeño pepper,* seeded

3 cloves garlic

2 teaspoons soy sauce or liquid aminos

1 tablespoon plus ¾ teaspoon salt, divided

½ cup peanut oil

1 package (about 12 ounces) uncooked soba noodles

Chopped fresh cilantro

Jalapeño peppers can sting and irritate the skin, so wear rubber gloves when handling peppers and do not touch your eyes.

1 Combine basil, ½ cup cilantro, ½ cup peanuts, jalapeño pepper, garlic, soy sauce and ¾ teaspoon salt in food processor; pulse until coarsely chopped. With motor running, drizzle in oil in thin, steady stream; process until well blended.

2 Bring large saucepan of water to a boil. Add remaining 1 tablespoon salt; stir until dissolved. Add noodles; return to a boil. Reduce heat to low. Cook 3 minutes or until tender. Drain and rinse under cold water to cool.

3 Place noodles in medium bowl; stir in pesto. Chop remaining ¼ cup peanuts; sprinkle over noodles. Garnish with chopped cilantro.

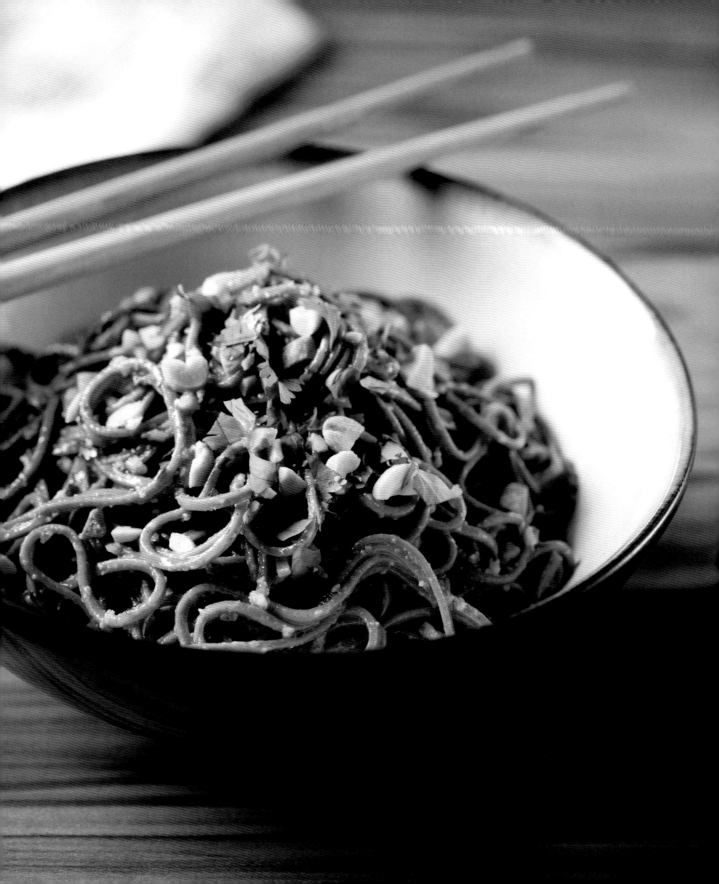

LENTIL
BOLOGNESE

  2 tablespoons olive oil

  1 onion, chopped

  1 carrot, chopped

  1 stalk celery, chopped

  2 cloves garlic, minced

  1 teaspoon salt

  ½ teaspoon dried oregano
     Pinch red pepper flakes

  3 tablespoons tomato paste

  ¼ cup dry white wine

  1 can (28 ounces) crushed
     tomatoes

  1 can (about 14 ounces) diced
     tomatoes

  1 cup dried lentils, rinsed

  1 portobello mushroom, gills
     removed, finely chopped

  1½ cups water or vegetable
     broth

     Hot cooked pasta

1 Heat oil in large saucepan over medium heat. Add onion, carrot and celery; cook and stir 10 minutes or until onion is lightly browned and carrots are softened.

2 Stir in garlic, salt, oregano and red pepper flakes. Add tomato paste; cook and stir 1 minute. Add wine; cook and stir until absorbed. Stir in crushed tomatoes, diced tomatoes, lentils, mushroom and water; bring to a simmer.

3 Reduce heat to medium; partially cover and simmer about 40 minutes or until lentils are tender, removing cover after 20 minutes. Serve over pasta.

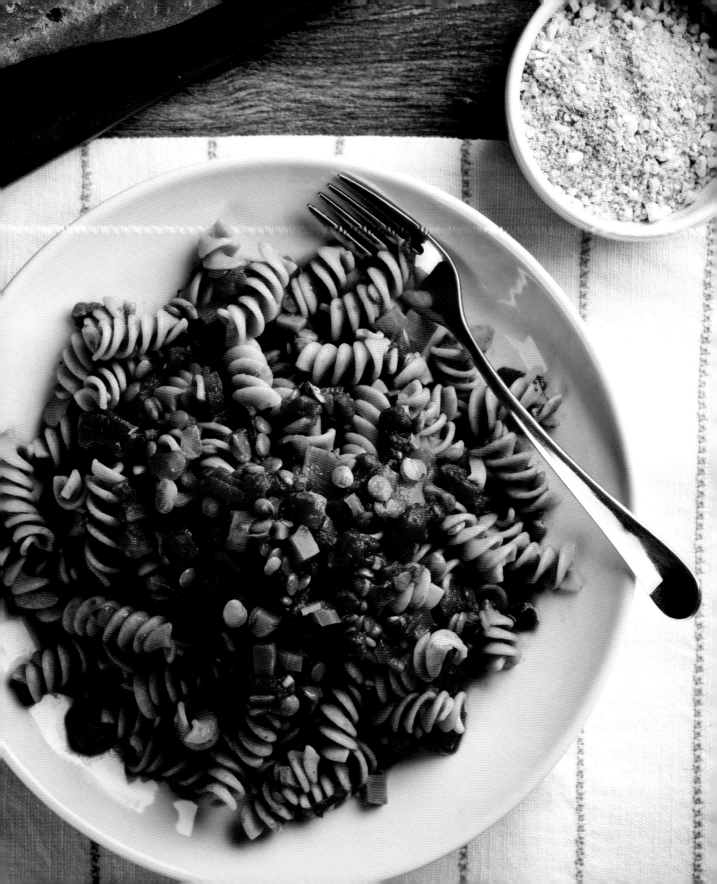

PORK TENDERLOIN WITH CABBAGE AND LEEKS

MAKES 4 SERVINGS

¼ cup olive oil, plus additional for pan

1 teaspoon salt

¾ teaspoon garlic powder

½ teaspoon dried thyme

½ teaspoon black pepper

1 pork tenderloin (about 1¼ pounds)

½ medium savoy cabbage, cored and cut into ¼-inch slices (about 6 cups)

1 small leek, cut in half lengthwise then cut crosswise into ¼-inch diagonal slices

1 to 2 teaspoons cider vinegar

1 Preheat oven to 450°F. Brush baking sheet with oil.

2 Combine salt, garlic powder, thyme and pepper in small bowl; mix well. Stir in ¼ cup oil until well blended. Brush pork with about 1 tablespoon oil mixture, turning to coat all sides.

3 Combine cabbage and leek in large bowl. Drizzle with remaining oil mixture; toss to coat. Spread on prepared baking sheet; top with pork.

4 Roast about 25 minutes or until pork is 145°F, stirring cabbage mixture halfway through cooking time. Remove pork to cutting board; tent with foil and let stand 10 minutes before slicing. Add vinegar to cabbage mixture; stir to blend.

Tip

If you can't find savoy cabbage, you can substitute regular green cabbage but it may take slightly longer to cook. If the cabbage is not crisp-tender when the pork is done, return the vegetables to the oven for 10 minutes or until crisp-tender.

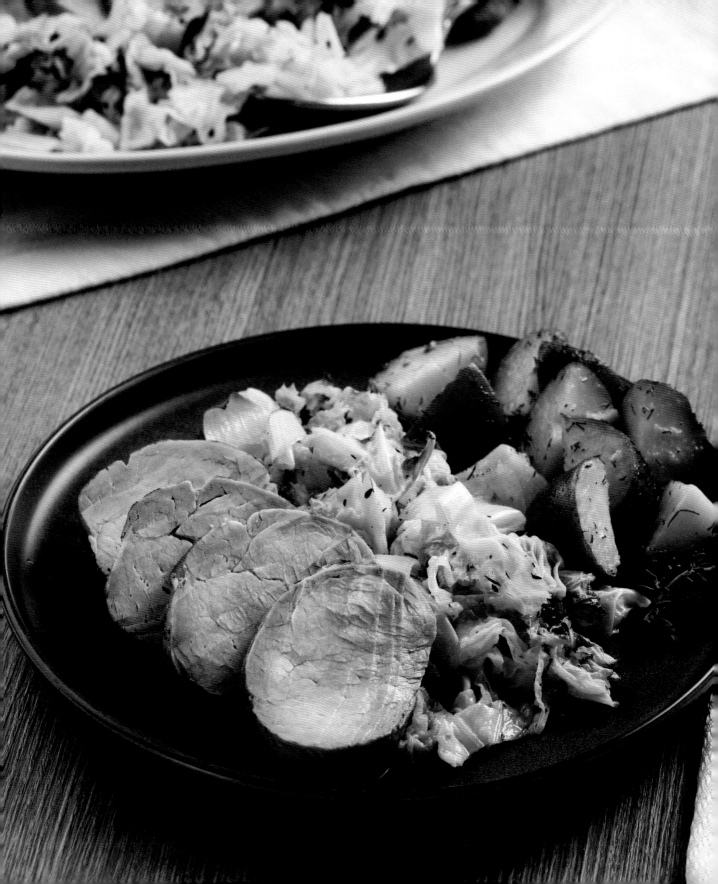

MUSHROOM TOFU BURGERS

MAKES 6 SERVINGS

3 tablespoons boiling water

1 tablespoon ground flaxseed

3 teaspoons olive oil, divided

1 package (8 ounces) cremini mushrooms, coarsely chopped

½ medium onion, coarsely chopped

1 clove garlic, minced

7 ounces extra firm tofu, crumbled and frozen

1 cup old-fashioned oats

⅓ cup finely chopped walnuts

½ teaspoon salt

½ teaspoon onion powder

¼ teaspoon dried thyme

6 English muffins, split and toasted

Optional toppings: lettuce, tomato and/or red onion slices

1 Combine boiling water and flaxseed in small bowl. Let stand until cool.

2 Heat 1 teaspoon oil in large nonstick skillet over medium heat. Add mushrooms, onion and garlic; cook and stir 10 minutes or until mushrooms have released most of their juices. Remove from heat; cool slightly.

3 Combine mushroom mixture, tofu, oats, walnuts, flaxseed mixture, salt, onion powder and thyme in food processor or blender; process until combined. (Some tofu pieces may remain). Shape mixture into 6 patties.

4 Heat 1 teaspoon oil in same skillet over medium-low heat. Working in batches, cook patties 5 minutes per side. Repeat with remaining 1 teaspoon oil and patties. Serve burgers on English muffins with lettuce, tomato and red onion, if desired.

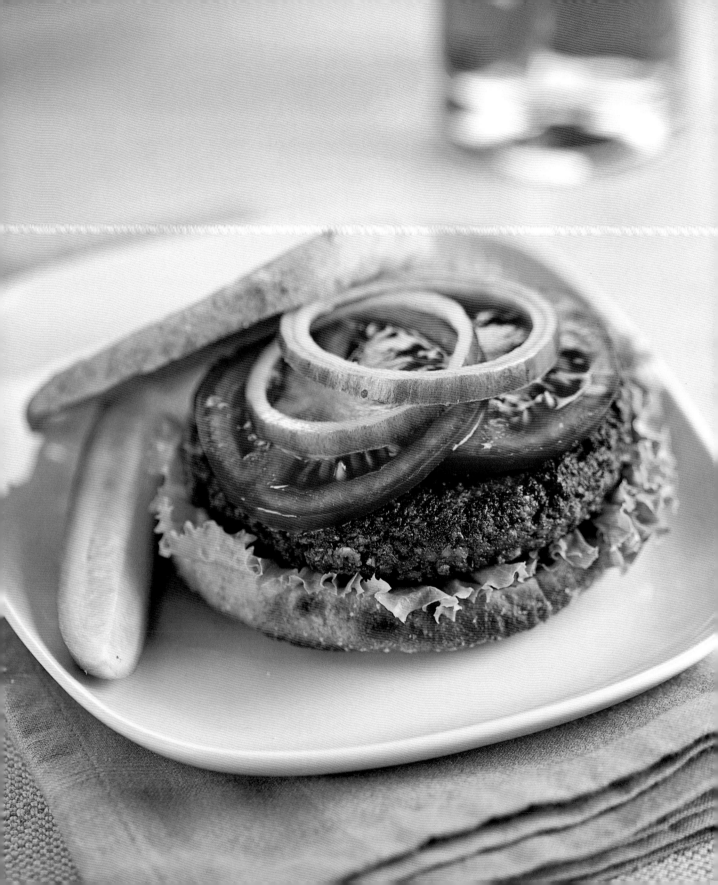

QUINOA PATTIES WITH ROASTED RED PEPPER SAUCE

MAKES 6 SERVINGS

1 cup uncooked quinoa

2 cups water

1 teaspoon salt, divided

¾ cup boiling water

¼ cup ground flaxseed

1 jar (12 ounces) roasted red peppers, drained

1 tablespoon balsamic vinegar

1 teaspoon lemon juice

1 teaspoon sugar

1 clove garlic

1 cup plain dry bread crumbs

⅓ cup nutritional yeast

2 tablespoons chopped fresh parsley

2 cloves garlic, minced

½ teaspoon Italian seasoning

1 to 2 tablespoons olive oil

1 Place quinoa in fine-mesh strainer; rinse well under cold running water.

2 Bring 2 cups water, quinoa and ½ teaspoon salt to a boil in medium saucepan over high heat. Reduce heat to low; cover and simmer 10 to 15 minutes or until quinoa is tender and water is absorbed. Cool slightly.

3 Combine boiling water and flaxseed in small bowl. Let stand until cool.

4 Meanwhile, blend roasted peppers, vinegar, lemon juice, sugar and garlic in blender or food processor until smooth. Set aside.

5 Combine quinoa, remaining ½ teaspoon salt, flaxseed mixture, bread crumbs, nutritional yeast, parsley, minced garlic and Italian seasoning in large bowl. Shape into 12 patties.

6 Heat 1 tablespoon oil in large skillet over medium heat. Add 6 patties; cook 5 to 7 minutes or until bottoms are browned. Flip patties; cook 5 to 7 minutes. Repeat with remaining patties, adding additional 1 tablespoon oil, if necessary. Serve patties with red pepper sauce.

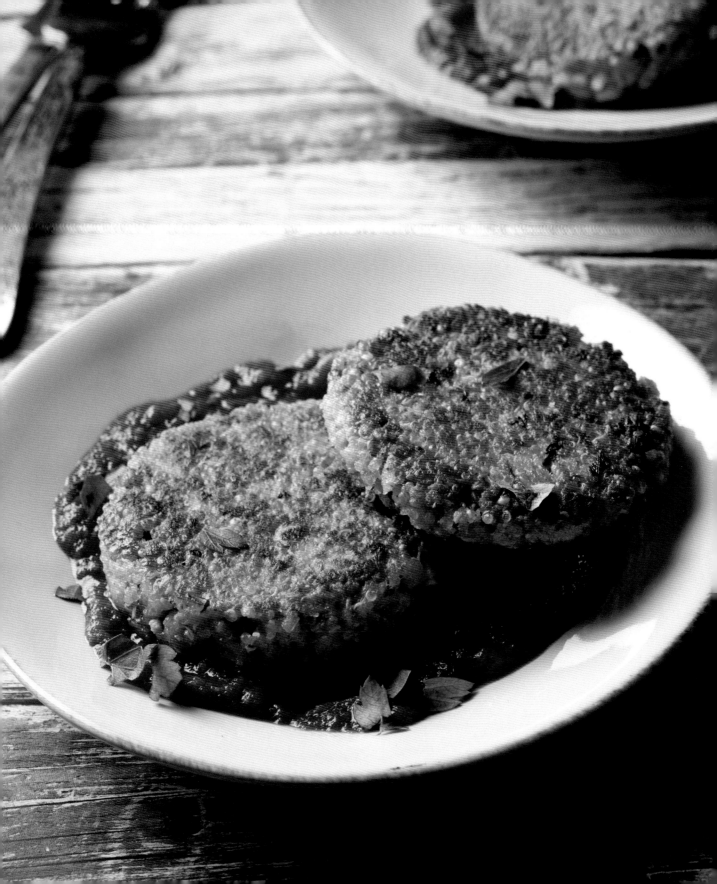

MEDITERRANEAN ROASTED VEGETABLE WRAPS

MAKES 4 SERVINGS

1 head cauliflower, cut into 1-inch florets

4 tablespoons olive oil, divided

2 teaspoons ras el hanout, 7-spice blend, shawarma blend or za'atar

1 teaspoon salt, divided

1 zucchini, quartered lengthwise and cut into ¼-inch pieces

1 yellow squash, quartered lengthwise and cut into ¼-inch pieces

½ red onion, thinly sliced

¼ cup red pepper sauce (avjar)

4 large thin pitas or lavash (10 inches)

4 ounces feta cheese, crumbled

1 cup chickpeas

¼ cup diced tomatoes

¼ cup minced fresh parsley

¼ cup diced cucumber (optional)

2 teaspoons vegetable oil

1 Preheat oven to 400°F. Combine cauliflower, 2 tablespoons olive oil, ras el hanout and ½ teaspoon salt in large bowl; toss to coat. Spread on half of sheet pan. Combine zucchini, yellow squash, onion, remaining 2 tablespoons olive oil and ½ teaspoon salt in same bowl; toss to coat. Spread on other side of sheet pan. Roast 25 minutes or until vegetables are browned and tender, stirring once. Remove from oven; cool slightly.

2 Spread 1 tablespoon red pepper sauce on 1 pita. Top with one fourth of vegetables, feta cheese, chickpeas, tomatoes, parsley and cucumber, if desired. Fold two sides over filling; roll up into burrito shape. Repeat with remaining ingredients.

3 Heat 1 teaspoon vegetable oil in large skillet over medium-high heat. Add 2 wraps, seam sides down; cook 1 minute or until browned. Turn and cook other side until browned. Repeat with remaining vegetable oil and wraps. Cut in half to serve.

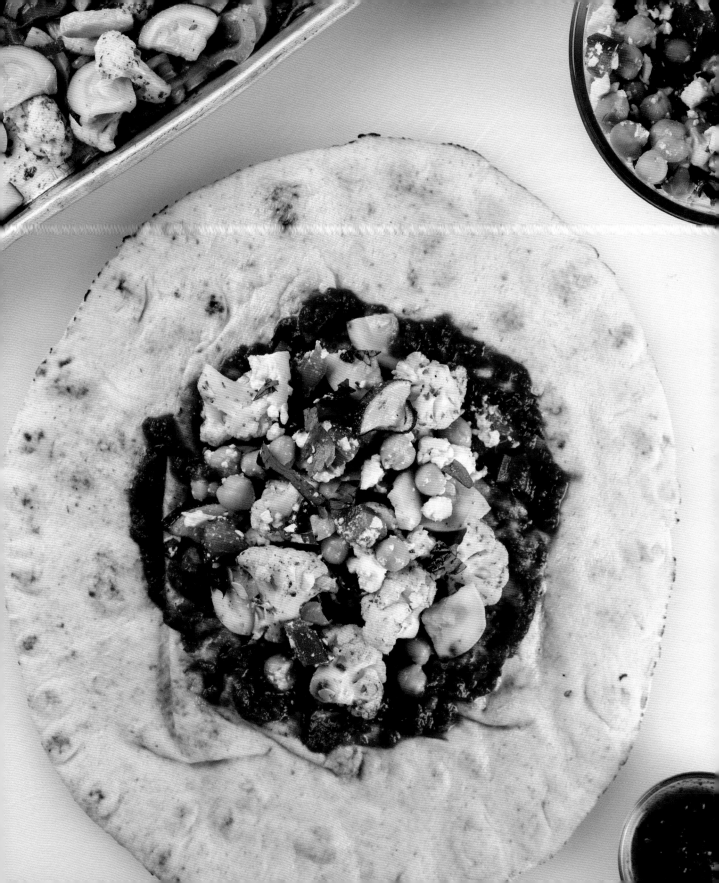

CHICKEN WITH QUINOA SALAD

MAKES 6 SERVINGS

1 cup uncooked tricolor quinoa

2 cups water

2½ teaspoons salt, divided

1 pint cherry tomatoes, halved

1 cucumber, quartered lengthwise and thinly sliced

4 boneless skinless chicken breasts (about 4 ounces each)

¾ teaspoon black pepper, divided

5 tablespoons extra virgin olive oil, divided

3 tablespoons fresh lemon juice

1 yellow or red bell pepper, chopped

½ cup minced fresh parsley

1 Rinse quinoa in fine-mesh strainer under cold running water. Combine 2 cups water, quinoa and 1 teaspoon salt in medium saucepan. Bring to a boil over high heat. Reduce heat to low; cover and simmer 10 to 15 minutes or until quinoa is tender and water is absorbed. Transfer to large bowl; cool to room temperature.

2 Meanwhile, combine tomatoes, cucumber and 1 teaspoon salt in medium bowl. Let stand 20 minutes.

3 Season chicken with remaining ½ teaspoon salt and ½ teaspoon black pepper.

4 Heat 1 tablespoon oil in large skillet over medium-high heat. Cook chicken about 5 minutes per side or until lightly browned and no longer pink in center. Remove to plate; keep warm.

5 Stir cucumbers, tomatoes and any accumulated juices into quinoa. Whisk remaining 4 tablespoons oil, lemon juice and remaining ¼ teaspoon black pepper in small bowl until well blended. Stir into quinoa mixture. Add bell pepper and parsley; mix until well blended. Taste and season with additional salt and pepper, if desired.

6 Slice chicken. Serve over quinoa salad.

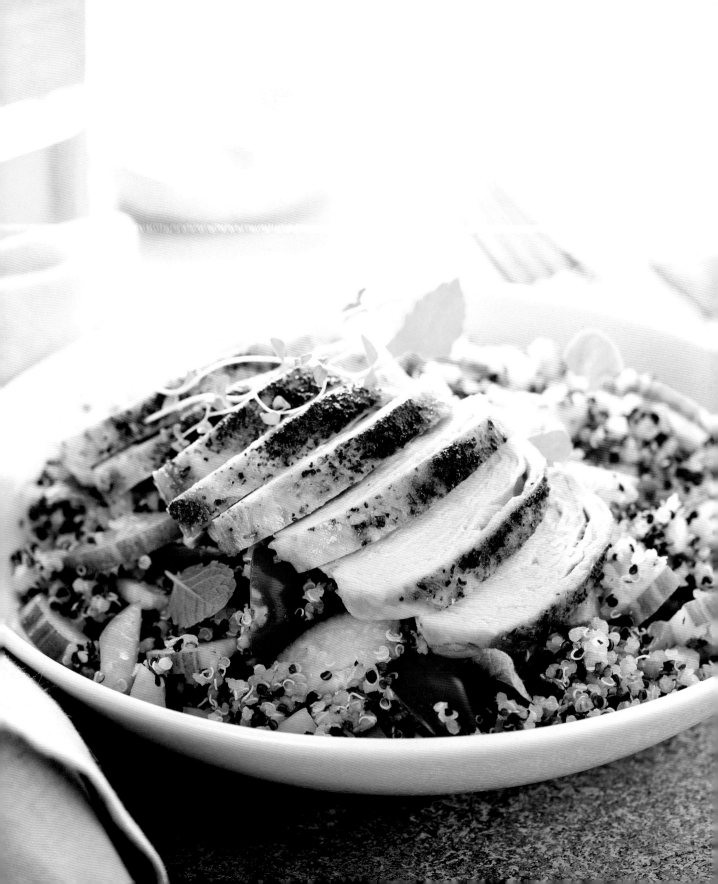

CHICKPEA BURGERS

3 tablespoons boiling water

1 tablespoon ground flaxseed

1 can (about 15 ounces) chickpeas, rinsed and drained

⅓ cup chopped carrots

⅓ cup panko bread crumbs

¼ cup chopped fresh parsley

¼ cup chopped onion

1 teaspoon minced garlic

1 teaspoon grated lemon peel

½ teaspoon salt

½ teaspoon black pepper

2 tablespoons vegetable or canola oil

4 whole grain hamburger buns

   Tomato slices, lettuce leaves and salsa (optional)

1 Combine boiling water and flaxseed in small bowl. Let stand until cool; refrigerate until ready to use.

2 Place chickpeas, carrots, panko, parsley, onion, garlic, lemon peel, salt and pepper in food processor; process until blended. Add flaxseed mixture; pulse until blended. Shape mixture into 4 patties.

3 Heat 1 tablespoon oil in large nonstick skillet over medium heat. Add patties; cook 4 to 5 minutes or until bottoms are browned. Add remaining 1 tablespoon to skillet; flip patties and cook 4 to 5 minutes or until browned. Serve burgers on buns with tomato, lettuce and salsa, if desired.

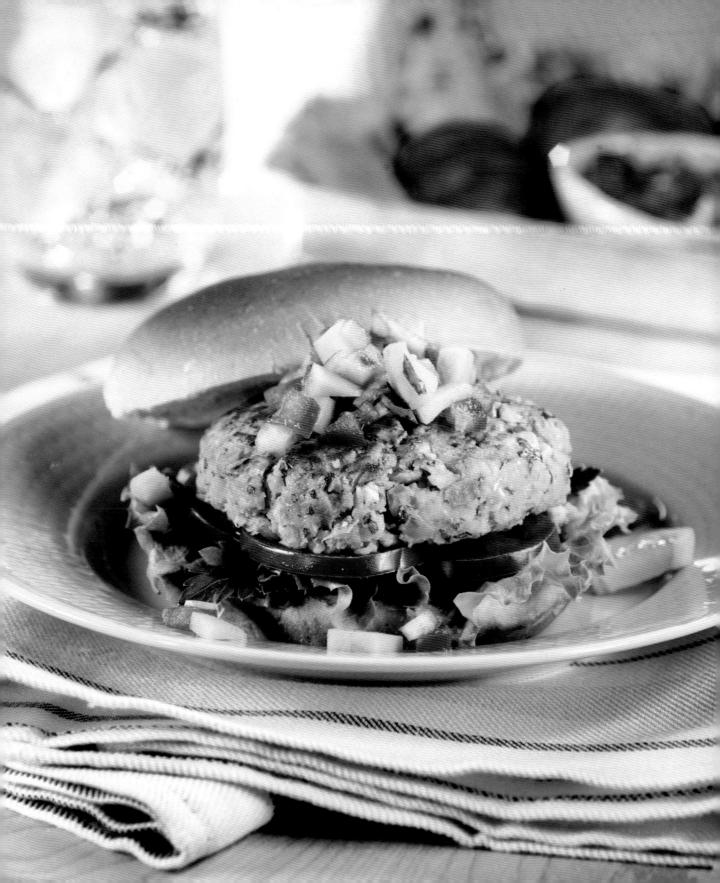

ORZO
SPINACH PIE

MAKES 4 SERVINGS

⅔ cup uncooked orzo

1 cup fat-free (skim) milk

3 egg whites

¼ teaspoon salt (optional)

⅛ teaspoon ground nutmeg

⅛ teaspoon black pepper

1 package (10 ounces) frozen
   chopped spinach, thawed
   and pressed dry

4 tablespoons grated
   Parmesan cheese, divided

¾ cup fresh whole wheat
   bread crumbs*

1 tablespoon unsalted butter,
   melted

*To make fresh bread crumbs, tear
1½ slices bread into pieces; process
in food processor until coarse
crumbs form.*

1 Preheat oven to 375°F. Spray 9-inch pie plate with
nonstick cooking spray.

2 Cook orzo according to package directions, omitting
any salt. Drain.

3 Whisk milk, egg whites, salt, if desired, nutmeg
and pepper in large bowl until well blended. Stir in
spinach and 2 tablespoons Parmesan cheese. Add
orzo; gently mix. Spoon evenly into prepared pie
plate.

4 Combine bread crumbs and remaining 2 tablespoons
Parmesan cheese in small bowl. Stir in butter.
Sprinkle evenly over spinach mixture.

5 Bake 20 minutes or until topping is golden brown
and center is set. Let stand 5 minutes before serving.

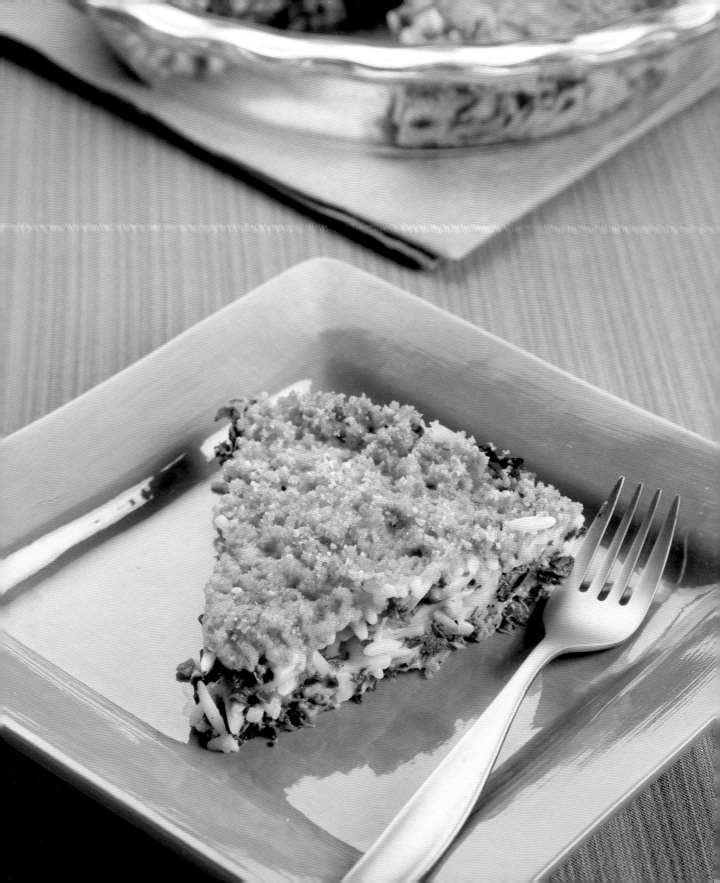

SHRIMP CAPRESE PASTA

MAKES 4 SERVINGS

1 cup uncooked whole wheat penne

2 teaspoons olive oil

2 cups coarsely chopped grape tomatoes

4 tablespoons chopped fresh basil, divided

1 tablespoon balsamic vinegar

2 cloves garlic, minced

¼ teaspoon salt

⅛ teaspoon red pepper flakes

8 ounces medium raw shrimp, peeled and deveined (with tails on)

1 cup grape tomatoes, halved

2 ounces fresh mozzarella pearls

1 Cook pasta according to package directions, omitting salt. Drain, reserving ½ cup cooking water. Set aside.

2 Heat oil in large skillet over medium heat. Add 2 cups chopped tomatoes, reserved ½ cup pasta water, 2 tablespoons basil, vinegar, garlic, salt and red pepper flakes. Cook and stir 10 minutes or until tomatoes begin to soften.

3 Add shrimp and 1 cup halved tomatoes to skillet; cook and stir 5 minutes or until shrimp turn pink and opaque. Add pasta; cook until heated through.

4 Divide mixture evenly among 4 bowls. Top evenly with cheese and remaining 2 tablespoons basil.

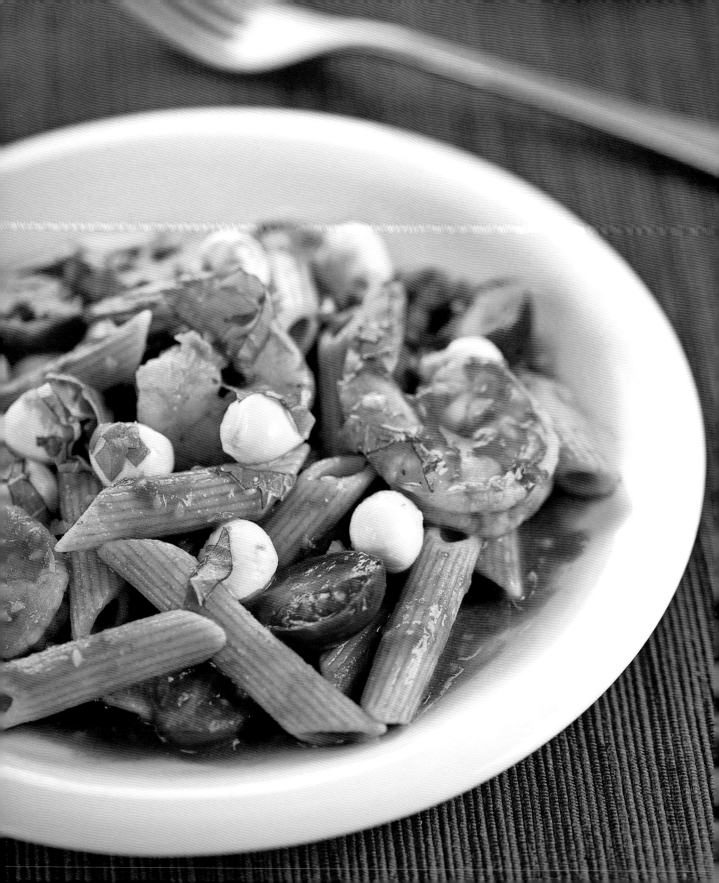

GRILLED RASPBERRY-THYME CHICKEN

MAKES 4 SERVINGS

4   boneless skinless chicken breasts (about 4 ounces each)

3   tablespoons plus 1 teaspoon red raspberry preserves, divided

1   tablespoon lemon juice

2   teaspoons reduced-sodium soy sauce, divided

¾   teaspoon grated lemon peel

¾   teaspoon dried thyme

2   tablespoons rice wine vinegar

2   teaspoons canola or vegetable oil

¾   pound fresh spinach, stemmed and torn

1   small cantaloupe, peeled and thinly sliced

6   ounces fresh raspberries

1 Place chicken in large resealable food storage bag. Blend 2 tablespoons raspberry preserves, lemon juice, 1 teaspoon soy sauce, lemon peel and thyme in small cup; pour into bag over chicken. Seal bag securely; turn bag several times to coat chicken with marinade. Refrigerate 1 hour.

2 For dressing, combine vinegar, remaining 4 teaspoons raspberry preserves, oil and remaining 1 teaspoon soy sauce in small jar with tight-fitting lid. Shake well; set aside.

3 Prepare grill for direct cooking over medium-high heat.* Arrange spinach, cantaloupe and raspberries on serving platter. Cover with plastic wrap; refrigerate until ready to use.

4 Remove chicken from marinade; reserve marinade. Grill 5 minutes. Brush top of chicken with marinade; discard remaining marinade. Turn chicken; grill 5 minutes or until no longer pink in center. Cut each breast diagonally into thin slices. Drizzle dressing over spinach and fruit; arrange chicken on top.

Chicken may be broiled instead of grilled. To broil, place chicken on rack in broiler pan. Cook 4 to 5 inches from heat 6 minutes. Turn chicken over; brush with reserved marinade. Cook 6 to 8 minutes longer or until juices run clear and chicken is no longer pink in center.

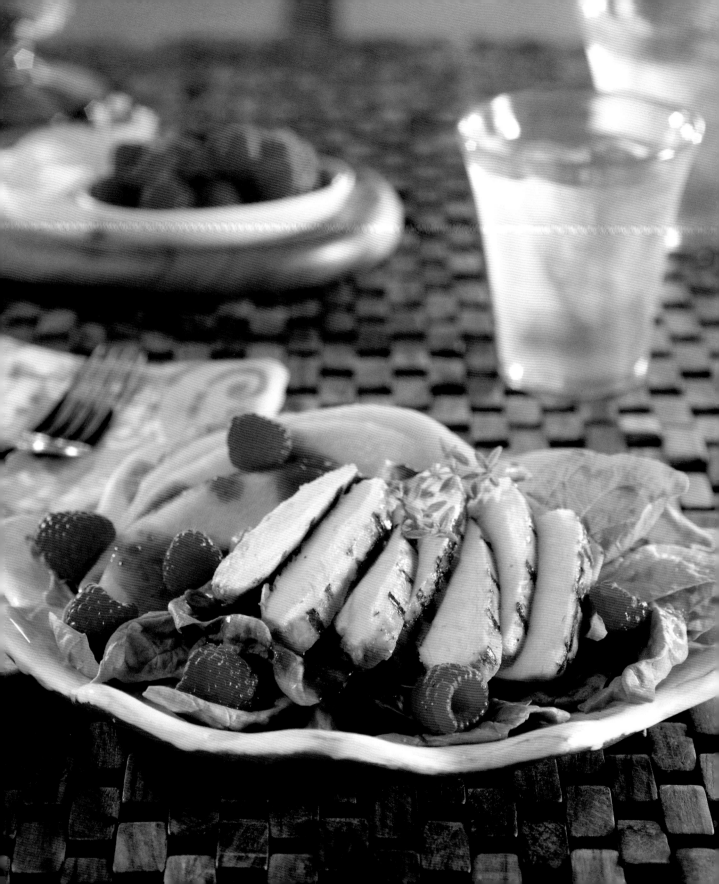

KALE & MUSHROOM STUFFED CHICKEN BREASTS

MAKES 4 SERVINGS

3 teaspoons olive oil, divided

1 cup coarsely chopped mushrooms

2 cups thinly sliced kale

1 tablespoon fresh lemon juice

½ teaspoon salt, divided

4 boneless skinless chicken breasts (about 4 ounces each)

¼ cup (1 ounce) crumbled feta cheese

¼ teaspoon black pepper

1 Heat 1 teaspoon oil in large skillet over medium-high heat. Add mushrooms; cook and stir 5 minutes or until mushrooms begin to brown. Add kale; cook and stir 8 minutes or until wilted. Sprinkle with lemon juice and ¼ teaspoon salt. Remove to small bowl. Let stand 5 to 10 minutes to cool slightly.

2 Meanwhile, place each chicken breast between sheets of plastic wrap. Pound with meat mallet or rolling pin to about ½-inch thickness.

3 Gently stir feta cheese into mushroom and kale mixture. Spoon ¼ cup mixture down center of each chicken breast. Roll up to enclose filling; secure with toothpicks. Sprinkle with remaining ¼ teaspoon salt and pepper.

4 Wipe out same skillet with paper towels. Add remaining 2 teaspoons oil to skillet; heat over medium heat. Add chicken; brown on all sides. Cover and cook 5 minutes per side or until no longer pink. Remove toothpicks before serving.

Serving Suggestion

Serve this flavorful entrée with a fresh salad or summer vegetables.

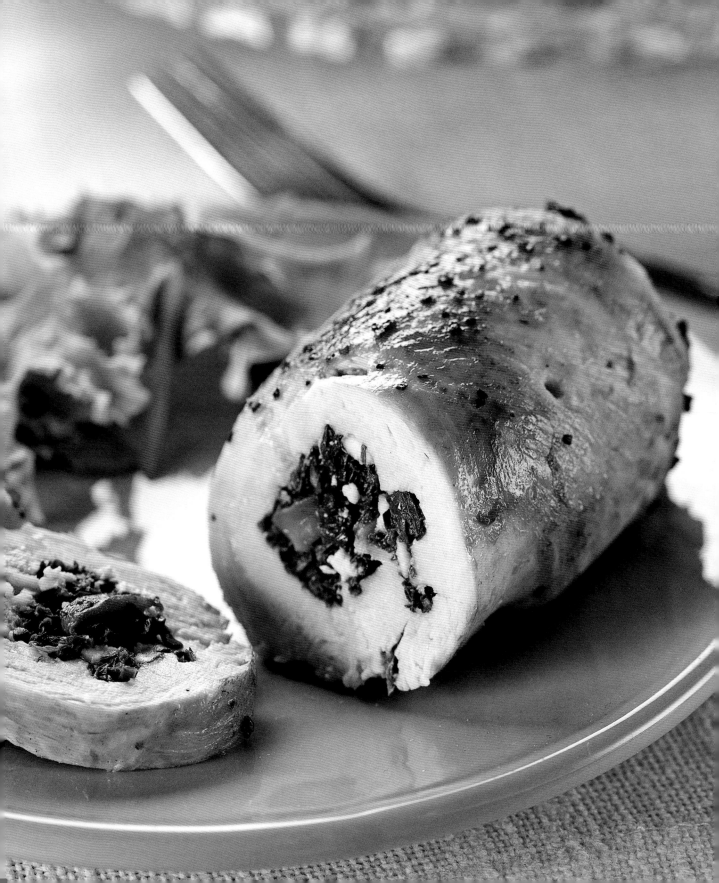

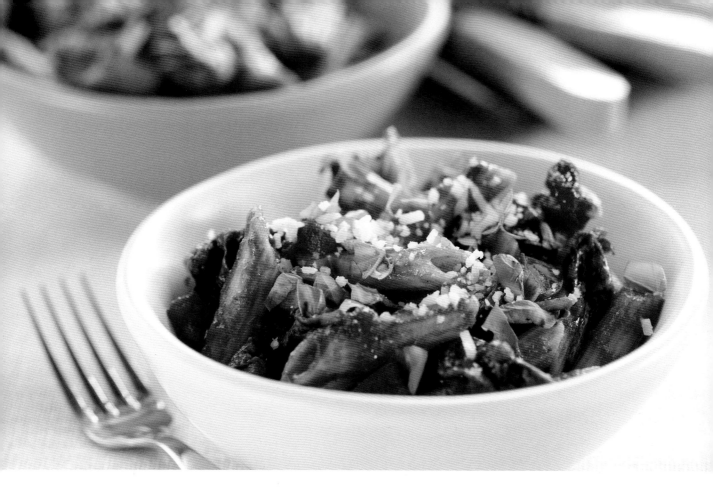

PENNE PASTA WITH CHUNKY TOMATO SAUCE AND SPINACH

MAKES 8 SERVINGS

8 ounces uncooked multigrain penne pasta

2 cups spicy marinara sauce

1 large ripe tomato, chopped (about 1½ cups)

4 cups packed baby spinach or torn spinach leaves (4 ounces)

¼ cup grated Parmesan cheese

¼ cup chopped fresh basil

1 Cook pasta according to package directions, omitting salt.

2 Meanwhile, heat marinara sauce and tomato in medium saucepan over medium heat 3 to 4 minutes or until hot and bubbly, stirring occasionally. Remove from heat; stir in spinach.

3 Drain pasta; return to saucepan. Add sauce; toss to combine. Divide evenly among 8 serving bowls; top with Parmesan cheese and basil.

EGGPLANT RIGATONI

8 ounces uncooked whole wheat rigatoni pasta

2 tablespoons olive oil, divided

2 medium eggplant, peeled and cut into 1-inch cubes

Salt and black pepper

½ cup (2 ounces) herb goat cheese

1 Cook pasta according to package directions. Reserve 1 cup cooking water; drain.

2 Heat 1 tablespoon oil in large nonstick skillet over medium heat. Add eggplant; cook and stir 20 minutes or until eggplant is soft and golden brown.

3 Add reserved cooking water to eggplant; stir well. Add pasta, remaining 1 tablespoon oil, salt and pepper. Toss to combine; cook until heated through.

4 Crumble goat cheese over pasta.

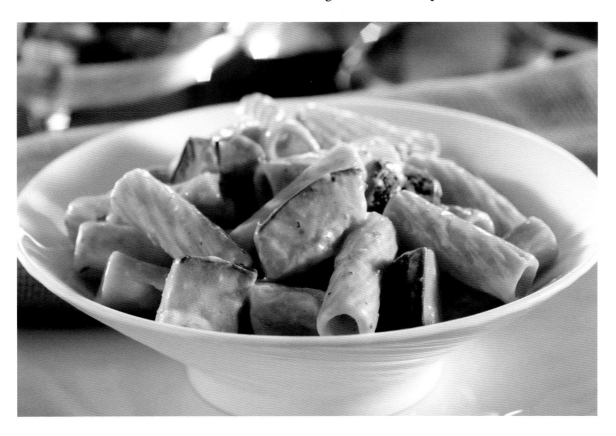

TURKEY LETTUCE WRAPS

**MAKES 12 WRAPS
(ABOUT 6 SERVINGS)**

1 teaspoon dark sesame oil

1 pound extra-lean ground turkey

½ cup sliced green onions

2 tablespoons minced fresh ginger

1 can (8 ounces) water chestnuts, chopped

1 teaspoon reduced-sodium soy sauce

¼ cup chopped fresh cilantro

12 large lettuce leaves

Chopped fresh mint and/ or chopped peanuts (optional)

1 Heat oil in large skillet over medium-high heat. Add turkey, green onions and ginger; cook 6 to 8 minutes, stirring to break up meat.

2 Add water chestnuts and soy sauce to skillet; cook 3 minutes or until turkey is no longer pink. Remove from heat; stir in cilantro.

3 Spoon ¼ cup turkey mixture onto each lettuce leaf. Top with chopped mint and/or peanuts, if desired. Roll up to enclose filling.

Variations

Use turkey mixture as a salad topping or substitute the lettuce leaves with corn tortillas.

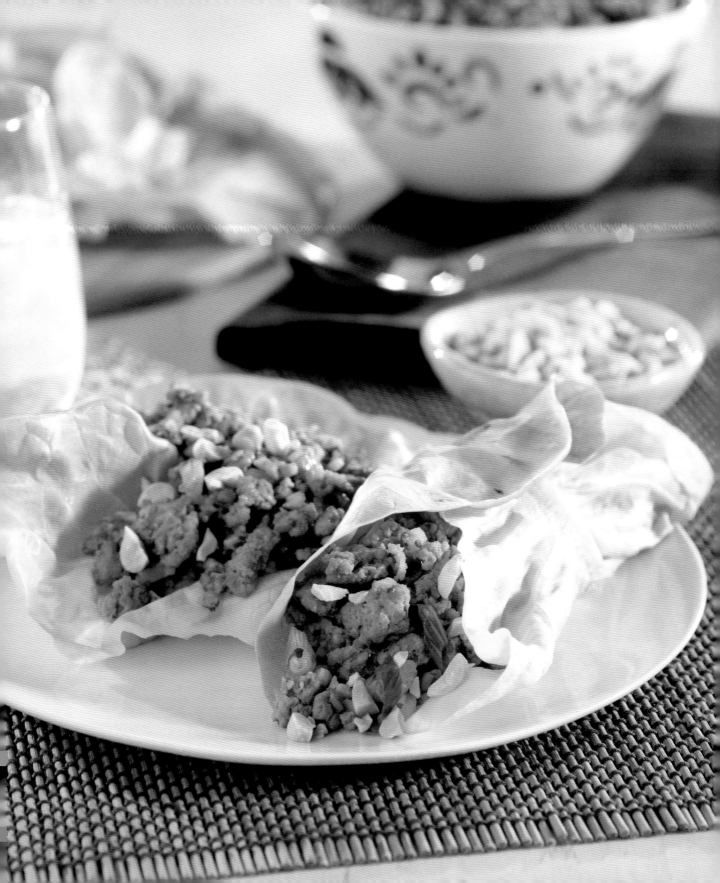

EGGPLANT PARMESAN

MAKES 4 SERVINGS

2 egg whites

2 tablespoons water

6 tablespoons seasoned dry bread crumbs

2 tablespoons plus ¼ cup grated Parmesan cheese, divided

1 large eggplant, peeled and cut into 12 round slices

2 teaspoons olive oil

1 small onion, diced

1 clove garlic, minced

2 cans (about 14 ounces each) diced tomatoes

½ teaspoon dried basil

½ teaspoon dried oregano

½ cup (2 ounces) shredded part-skim mozzarella cheese

1 Preheat oven to 350°F. Spray 15×10×1-inch jelly-roll pan with nonstick cooking spray.

2 Whisk egg whites and water in shallow dish. Combine bread crumbs and 2 tablespoons Parmesan cheese in another shallow dish. Dip eggplant slices in egg white mixture, then in bread crumb mixture, pressing lightly to adhere crumbs.

3 Place eggplant slices in single layer in prepared pan. Bake 25 to 30 minutes or until bottoms are browned. Turn slices; bake 15 to 20 minutes or until well browned and tender.

4 Meanwhile, heat oil in medium nonstick skillet over medium-high heat. Add onion; cook and stir 5 minutes or until softened. Add garlic; cook and stir 1 minute. Stir in tomatoes, basil and oregano; bring to a boil. Reduce heat to low; simmer 15 to 20 minutes or until sauce is thickened, stirring occasionally.

5 Spray 13×9-inch baking dish with cooking spray. Spread sauce in dish. Arrange eggplant slices in single layer on top of sauce. Sprinkle with mozzarella cheese and remaining ¼ cup Parmesan cheese. Bake 15 to 20 minutes or until sauce is bubbly and cheese melts.

Tip

Cut eggplant slices ½ to ¼ inch thick for best results.

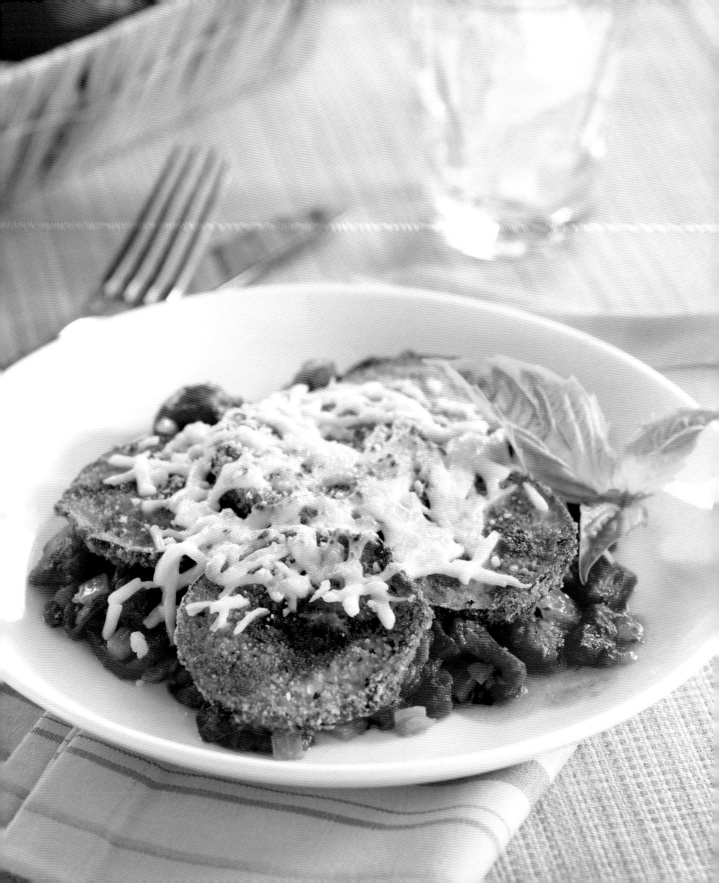

SPEEDY SPAGHETTI WITH SAUSAGE

MAKES 6 SERVINGS

12 ounces whole wheat spaghetti

8 ounces hot Italian turkey sausage, casing removed

1 cup chopped onion

3 cloves garlic, minced

1 can (28 ounces) crushed or puréed tomatoes, undrained

1 can (about 14 ounces) no-salt-added stewed tomatoes, undrained

1 teaspoon dried basil

¼ teaspoon red pepper flakes (optional)

1 large *or* 2 medium zucchini or yellow squash, cut into chunks

¼ cup grated Parmesan cheese

1 Cook spaghetti according to package directions, omitting salt. Drain and set aside.

2 Meanwhile, crumble sausage into large saucepan. Add onion and garlic. Cook over medium heat until sausage is no longer pink, stirring occasionally; drain if needed.

3 Add crushed tomatoes with juice, stewed tomatoes with juice, basil and red pepper flakes, if desired; bring to a simmer. Stir in zucchini; return to a simmer and cook, uncovered, 15 minutes or until zucchini is tender and sauce thickens, stirring occasionally.

4 Top cooked pasta with sauce; sprinkle with Parmesan cheese.

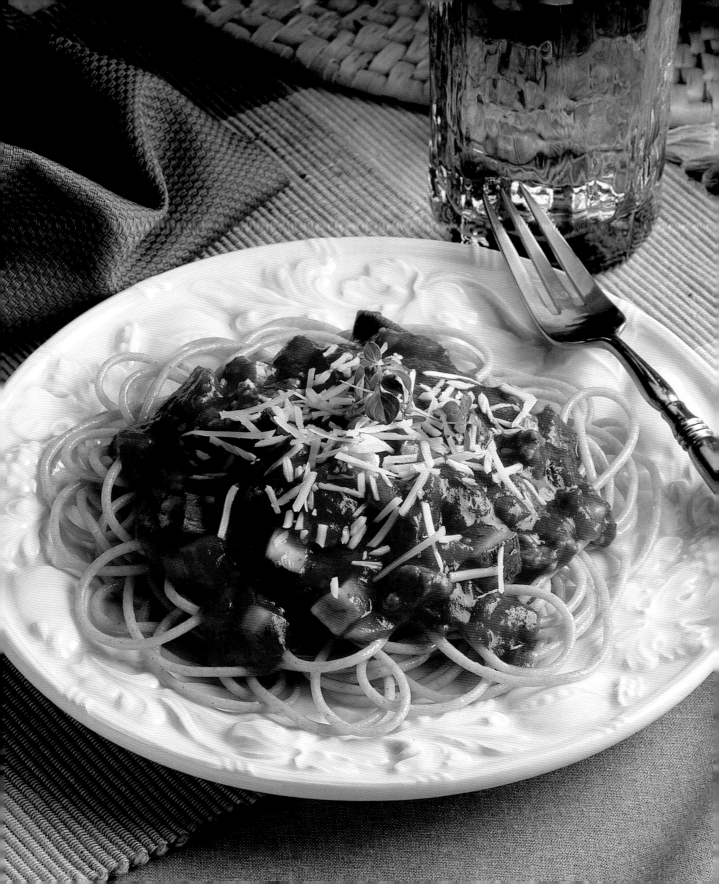

VEGETABLE-BEAN QUESADILLAS

MAKES 8 SERVINGS

1 tablespoon canola oil

1 cup sliced onion

1 can (about 15 ounces) black beans, rinsed and drained

1 cup sliced green bell pepper

1 cup sliced red bell pepper

½ teaspoon ground cumin

¼ teaspoon ground red pepper

8 (8-inch) whole grain tortillas

1 cup (4 ounces) shredded Cheddar cheese

Salsa and sour cream (optional)

1 Heat oil in large nonstick skillet over medium-high heat. Add onion; cook and stir 2 minutes or until translucent. Add beans, bell peppers, cumin and red pepper; cook and stir 3 minutes or until bell peppers are crisp-tender.

2 Heat medium nonstick skillet over medium heat. Place 1 tortilla in skillet. Spread about ⅓ cup vegetables on half of tortilla; sprinkle with 2 tablespoons cheese. Fold tortilla over filling and cook until light brown on bottom. Turn and brown other side. Fill and cook remaining tortillas. Cut into wedges. Serve with salsa and sour cream, if desired.

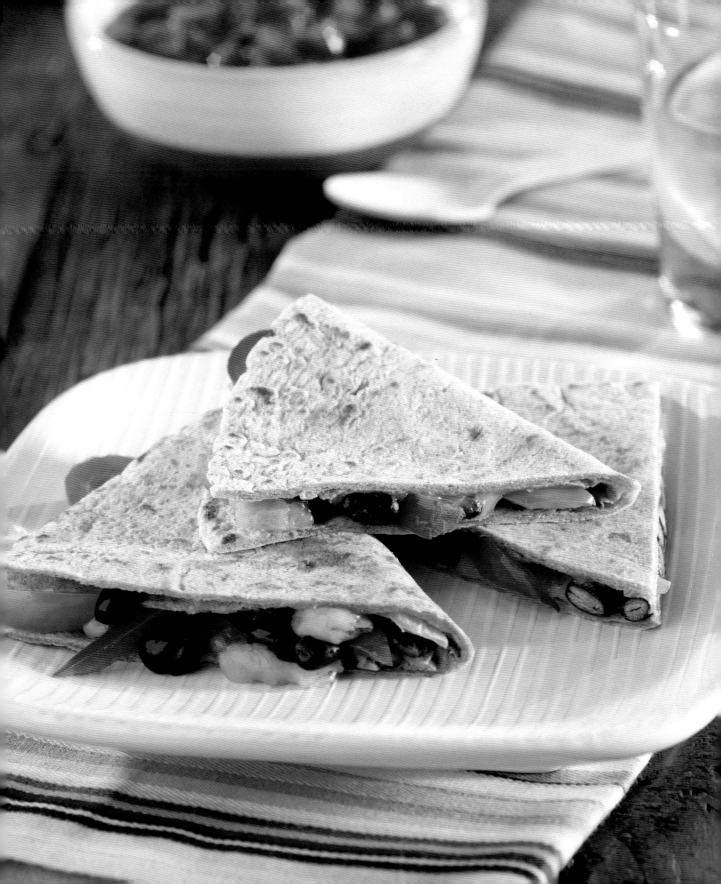

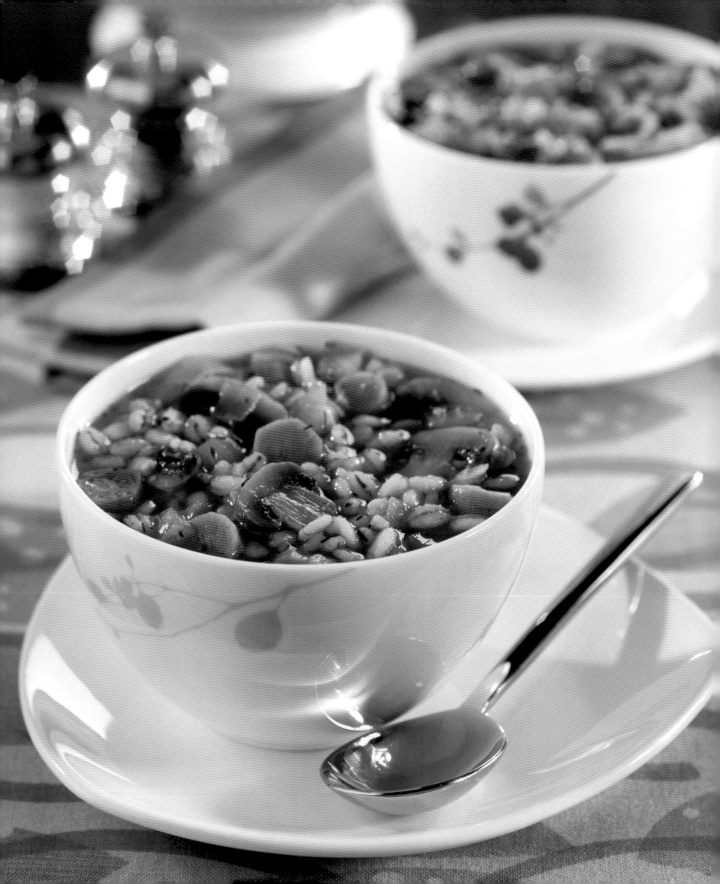

BEST BOWLS & SOUPS

MUSHROOM BARLEY SOUP

2 tablespoons olive oil

8 ounces sliced mushrooms

½ cup chopped onion

½ cup chopped carrots

1 clove garlic, minced

1 teaspoon dried thyme

¼ teaspoon black pepper

¼ cup dry white wine

4 cups chicken broth

¾ cup quick-cooking barley

1 Heat oil in large saucepan over medium-high heat. Add mushrooms, onion, carrots, garlic, thyme and pepper; cook and stir 6 to 8 minutes or until mushrooms begin to brown. Add wine, stirring to scrape up browned bits from bottom of saucepan.

2 Stir in broth; bring to a boil over high heat. Stir in barley. Reduce heat to low; simmer, partially covered, 15 minutes or until barley is tender.

Tips

For extra flavor, use a mix of button and baby bella mushrooms. For a vegetarian soup, substitute vegetable broth for the chicken broth.

CHICKEN BURRITO BOWLS

3 cloves garlic

½ medium red onion, coarsely chopped

2 tablespoons olive oil

1½ tablespoons adobo sauce (from small can of chipotle peppers in adobo)

1 tablespoon ancho chili powder

1½ teaspoons ground cumin

1 teaspoon salt

1 teaspoon dried oregano

½ teaspoon black pepper

½ cup water

1 pound boneless skinless chicken thighs

1⅓ cups cooked black beans

3 cups cooked white or brown rice

Optional toppings: guacamole, salsa, corn, shredded lettuce, shredded Monterey Jack cheese, lime wedges, sour cream, tortilla chips

1 With motor running, drop garlic cloves through feed tube of food processor; process until garlic is finely chopped. Add onion, oil, adobo sauce, chili powder, cumin, salt, oregano and pepper; process until well blended. Add water; process until smooth.

2 Place chicken in large resealable food storage bag. Add marinade; seal bag and turn to coat. Refrigerate at least 3 hours or overnight.

3 Remove chicken from refrigerator about 30 minutes before cooking. Prepare grill for direct cooking or preheat grill pan.* Grill chicken about 6 minutes per side or until cooked through (160°F). Remove to large plate; tent with foil. Let stand 10 minutes before chopping into ½-inch pieces.

4 Serve chicken and beans over rice with desired toppings.

*Or cook chicken in large skillet in 1 tablespoon olive oil over medium-high heat about 6 minutes per side or until browned and cooked through (160°F).

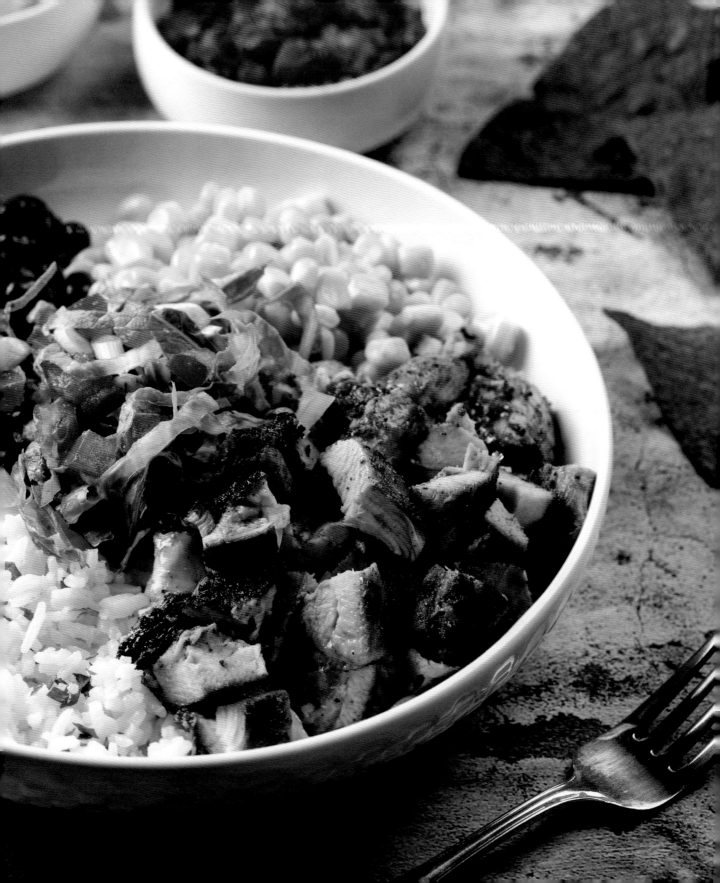

BLACK BEAN SOUP

2 tablespoons vegetable oil

1 cup diced onion

1 stalk celery, diced

2 carrots, diced

½ small green bell pepper, diced

4 cloves garlic, minced

4 cans (about 15 ounces each) black beans, rinsed and drained, divided

1 container (32 ounces) vegetable broth, divided

2 tablespoons cider vinegar

2 teaspoons chili powder

½ teaspoon salt

½ teaspoon ground red pepper

½ teaspoon ground cumin

¼ teaspoon liquid smoke

Optional toppings: sour cream, chopped green onions and shredded cheese

1 Heat oil in large saucepan or Dutch oven over medium-low heat. Add onion, celery, carrots, bell pepper and garlic; cook 10 minutes, stirring occasionally.

2 Combine half of beans and 1 cup broth in food processor or blender; process until smooth. Add to vegetables in saucepan.

3 Stir in remaining beans, remaining broth, vinegar, chili powder, salt, red pepper, cumin and liquid smoke; bring to a boil over high heat. Reduce heat to medium-low; cook 1 hour or until vegetables are tender and soup is thickened. Serve with desired toppings.

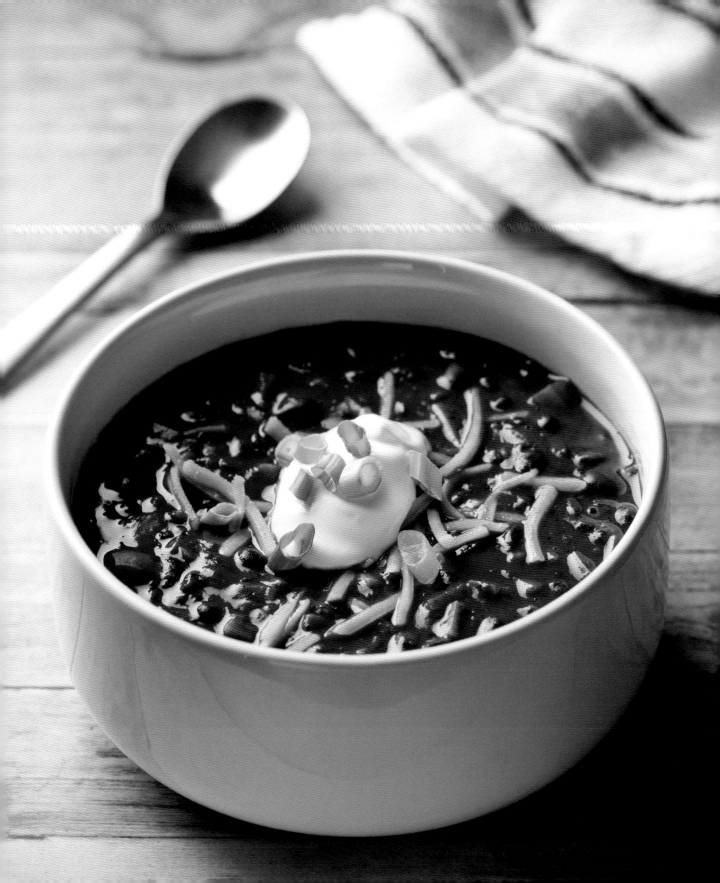

TOFU IN PURGATORY

MAKES 4 SERVINGS

- 2 tablespoons olive oil
- 1 large onion, chopped
- 2 cloves garlic, minced
- 2 tablespoons tomato paste
- 1 teaspoon salt
- 1 teaspoon ground cumin
- 1 teaspoon ground coriander
- ½ teaspoon smoked paprika
- 1 can (28 ounces) diced tomatoes
- Crispy Toast (recipe follows)
- 1 package (about 12 ounces) firm silken tofu, cut into 8 cubes
- Shredded fresh basil

1 Heat oil in large skillet over medium-high heat. Add onion; cook and stir 5 minutes or until softened. Add garlic, tomato paste, salt, cumin, coriander and paprika; cook and stir 1 minute.

2 Stir in tomatoes; bring to a simmer. Reduce heat to medium-low; cook 20 minutes, stirring occasionally. Meanwhile, prepare Crispy Toast.

3 Make 8 divots in sauce; add tofu cubes. Cover and cook 10 minutes to heat tofu. Scoop into bowls; garnish with basil and serve with toast.

Crispy Toast

Preheat oven to 400°F. Place 4 to 8 slices of whole grain, French, Italian or sourdough bread on baking sheet. Brush olive oil all over both sides of bread. Bake 8 to 10 minutes or until golden brown and crisp, turning once. Cut 2 garlic cloves in half; rub cut sides all over one side of each toast.

78

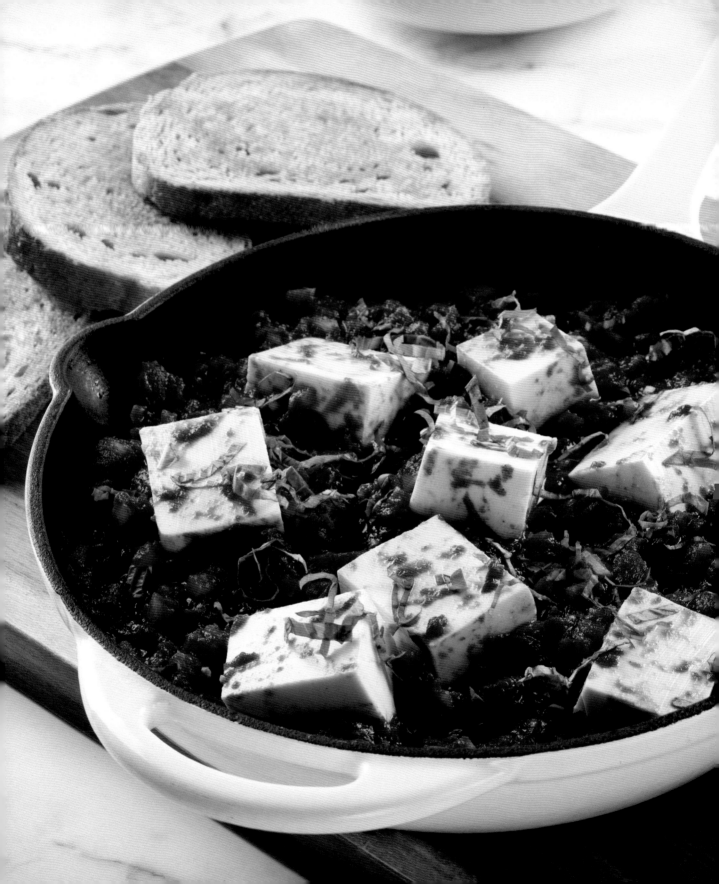

CHICKPEA TIKKA MASALA

1 tablespoon olive oil

1 onion, chopped

3 cloves garlic, minced

1 tablespoon minced fresh ginger *or* ginger paste

1 tablespoon garam masala

1 teaspoon ground cumin

1 teaspoon ground coriander

1 teaspoon salt

¼ teaspoon ground red pepper

2 cans (15 ounces each) chickpeas, drained

1 can (28 ounces) crushed tomatoes

1 can (about 13 ounces) coconut milk

1 package (about 12 ounces) firm silken tofu, drained and cut into 1-inch cubes

Hot cooked brown basmati rice

Chopped fresh cilantro

1 Heat oil in large saucepan over medium-high heat. Add onion; cook and stir 5 minutes or until translucent. Add garlic, ginger, garam masala, cumin, coriander, salt and red pepper; cook and stir 1 minute.

2 Stir in chickpeas, tomatoes and coconut milk; simmer 30 minutes or until thickened and chickpeas have softened slightly. Add tofu; stir gently. Cook 7 to 10 minutes or until tofu is heated through. Serve over rice; garnish with cilantro.

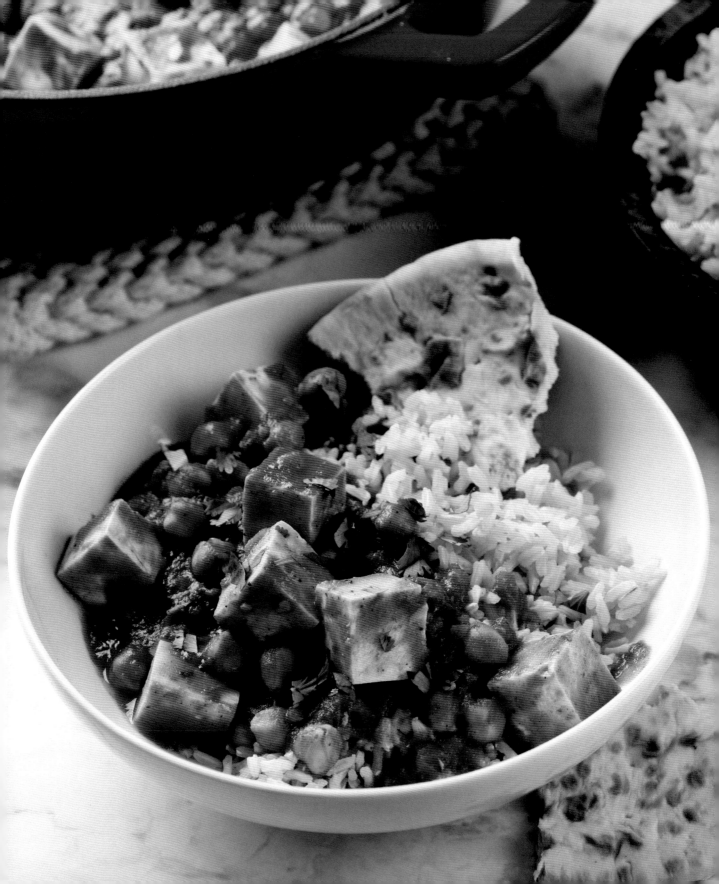

QUINOA BURRITO BOWLS

1 cup uncooked quinoa

2 cups water

2 tablespoons fresh lime juice, divided

¼ cup sour cream

2 teaspoons vegetable oil

1 small onion, diced

1 red bell pepper, diced

1 clove garlic, minced

½ cup canned black beans, rinsed and drained

½ cup thawed frozen corn

Shredded lettuce

1 Place quinoa in fine-mesh strainer; rinse well under cold running water. Bring 2 cups water to a boil in small saucepan; stir in quinoa. Reduce heat to low; cover and simmer 10 to 15 minutes or until quinoa is tender and water is absorbed. Stir in 1 tablespoon lime juice.

2 Combine sour cream and remaining 1 tablespoon lime juice in small bowl; set aside.

3 Meanwhile, heat oil in large skillet over medium heat. Add onion and bell pepper; cook and stir 5 minutes or until softened. Add garlic; cook 1 minute. Add black beans and corn; cook 3 to 5 minutes or until heated through.

4 Divide quinoa among serving bowls; top with black bean mixture, lettuce and sour cream mixture.

Note

This bowl makes a great packable lunch. Layer the quinoa mixture and bean mixture in glass food storage container with lid or glass jar. Pack lettuce and sour cream mixture separately. Heat quinoa and beans in the microwave until warm; top with lettuce and sour cream.

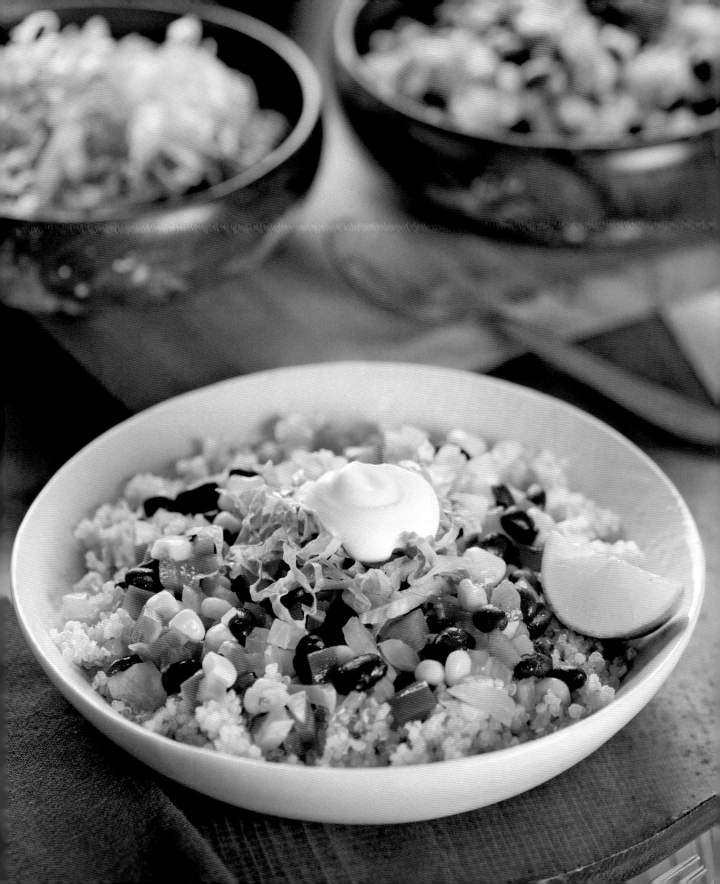

PEPPERY SICILIAN
CHICKEN SOUP

MAKES 8 TO 10 SERVINGS

2 tablespoons olive oil

1 onion, chopped

1 green bell pepper, chopped

3 stalks celery, chopped

3 carrots, chopped

3 cloves garlic, minced

1 tablespoon salt

3 containers (32 ounces each) chicken broth

2 pounds boneless skinless chicken breasts

1 can (28 ounces) diced tomatoes

2 baking potatoes, peeled and cut into ¼-inch pieces

1½ teaspoons ground white pepper*

1½ teaspoons ground black pepper

½ cup chopped fresh parsley

8 ounces uncooked ditalini pasta

Or substitute additional black pepper for the white pepper.

1 Heat oil in large saucepan or Dutch oven over medium heat. Stir in onion, bell pepper, celery and carrots. Reduce heat to medium-low; cover and cook 10 to 15 minutes or until vegetables are tender but not browned, stirring occasionally. Stir in garlic and salt; cover and cook 5 minutes.

2 Stir in broth, chicken, tomatoes, potatoes, white pepper and black pepper; bring to a boil. Reduce heat to low; cover and simmer 1 hour. Remove chicken to plate; set aside until cool enough to handle. Shred chicken and return to saucepan with parsley.

3 Meanwhile, cook pasta in medium saucepan of boiling salted water 7 minutes (or 1 minute less than package directs for al dente). Drain pasta; add to soup.

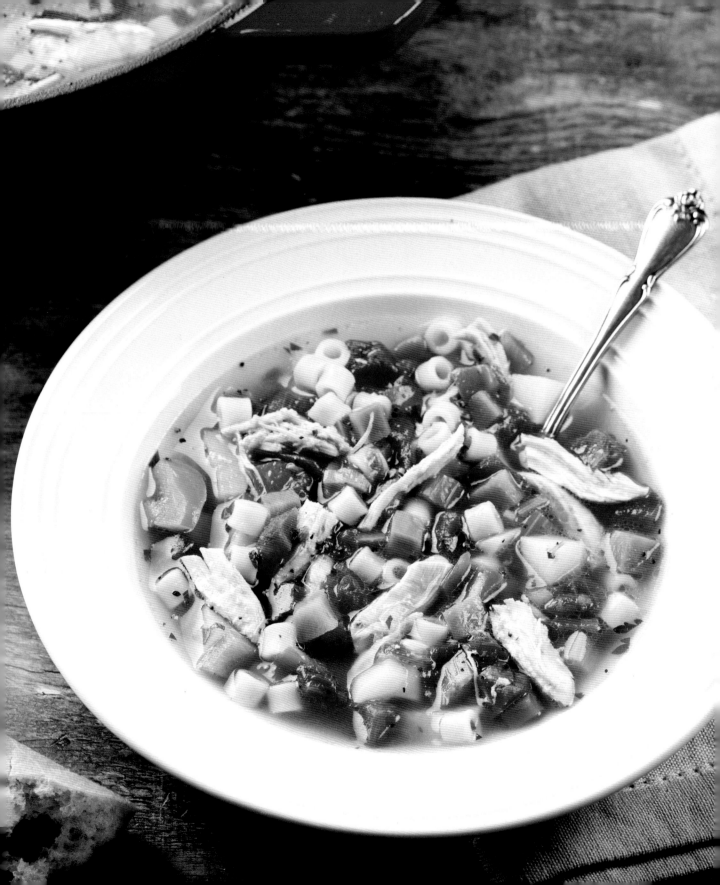

KOSHARI

4 cups water

1 cup uncooked white
   basmati rice, rinsed and
   drained

1 cup dried brown lentils,
   rinsed and sorted

3 teaspoons kosher salt,
   divided

1 teaspoon ground
   cinnamon, divided

½ teaspoon ground nutmeg,
   divided

1 cup uncooked elbow
   macaroni

2 tablespoons olive oil,
   divided

1 large onion, thinly sliced

1 large onion, diced

1 tablespoon minced garlic

1 teaspoon ground cumin

½ teaspoon ground coriander

¼ teaspoon red pepper flakes

¼ teaspoon black pepper

1 can (28 ounces) crushed
   tomatoes

2 teaspoons red wine vinegar

Slow Cooker Directions

1 Place water, rice, lentils, 2 teaspoons salt, ½ teaspoon cinnamon and ¼ teaspoon nutmeg in slow cooker. Cover; cook on HIGH 2 hours 30 minutes. Stir in macaroni. Cover; cook 30 minutes, stirring halfway through cooking time.

2 Meanwhile, heat 1 tablespoon oil in large skillet over medium-high heat. Add sliced onion; cook 12 minutes or until edges are dark brown and onion is softened. Remove onions to medium bowl, using slotted spoon. Season with ¼ teaspoon salt. Set aside.

3 Heat same skillet with remaining 1 tablespoon oil over medium heat. Add diced onion; cook 8 minutes or until softened. Add garlic, cumin, coriander, remaining ½ teaspoon cinnamon, red pepper flakes, black pepper and remaining ¼ teaspoon nutmeg; cook 30 seconds or until fragrant. Stir in tomatoes, vinegar and remaining ¾ teaspoon salt; cook 8 to 10 minutes or until thickened, stirring occasionally.

4 Fluff rice mixture lightly before scooping into individual bowls. Top each serving evenly with tomato sauce and reserved onions.

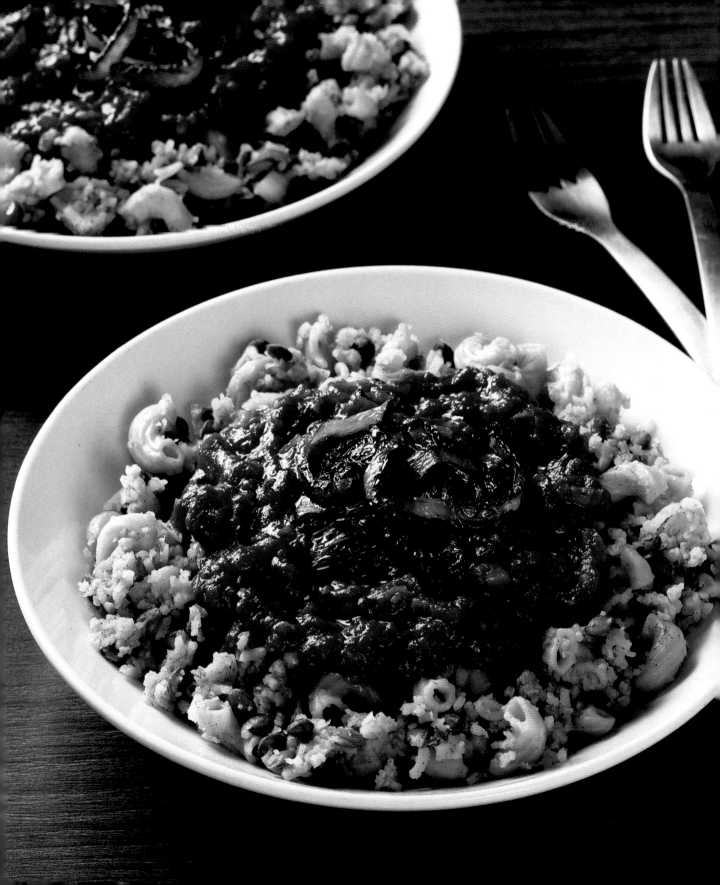

VEGETARIAN QUINOA CHILI

MAKES 4 TO 6 SERVINGS

2 tablespoons vegetable oil

1 large onion, chopped

1 red bell pepper, chopped

1 large carrot, diced

1 stalk celery, diced

1 jalapeño pepper,* seeded and finely chopped

1 tablespoon minced garlic

1 tablespoon chili powder

2 teaspoons ground cumin

1 teaspoon kosher salt (optional)

1 can (28 ounces) crushed tomatoes

1 can (about 15 ounces) kidney beans, rinsed and drained

1 cup water

1 cup fresh or frozen corn

½ cup uncooked quinoa, rinsed well

Optional toppings: diced avocado, shredded Cheddar cheese and sliced green onions

*Jalapeño peppers can sting and irritate the skin, so wear rubber gloves when handling peppers and do not touch your eyes.

1 Heat oil in large saucepan over medium-high heat. Add onion, bell pepper, carrot and celery; cook 10 minutes or until vegetables are softened, stirring occasionally. Add jalapeño pepper, garlic, chili powder, cumin and salt, if desired; cook 1 minute or until fragrant.

2 Add tomatoes, beans, water, corn and quinoa; bring to a boil. Reduce heat to low; cover and simmer 1 hour, stirring occasionally.

3 Spoon into bowls; top as desired.

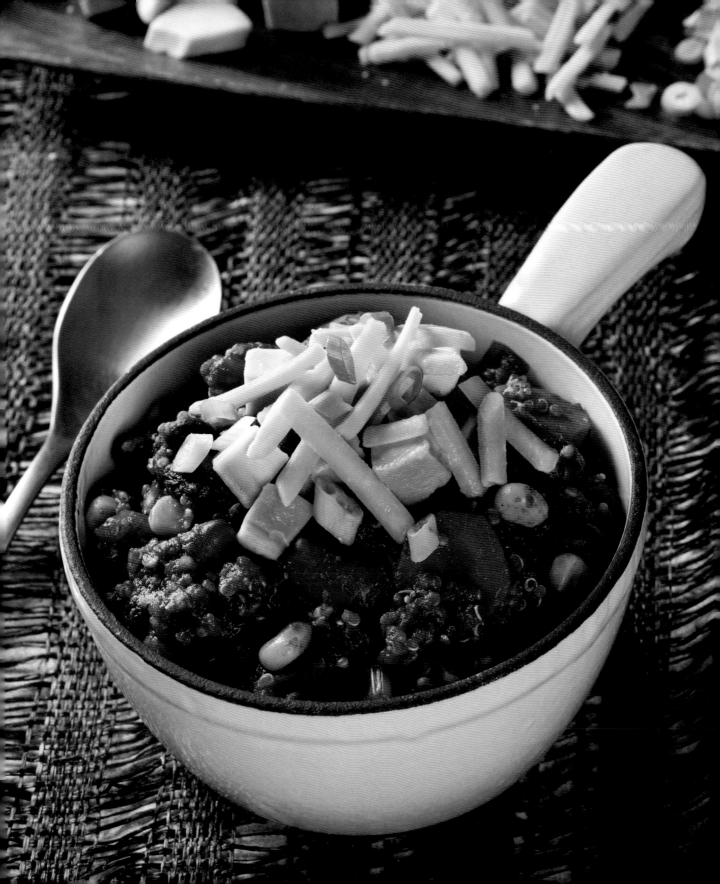

SPICY LENTIL AND PASTA SOUP

- 2 medium onions, thinly sliced
- ½ cup chopped carrot
- ½ cup chopped celery
- ½ cup chopped peeled turnip
- 1 small jalapeño pepper,* finely chopped
- 2 cups water
- 2 cans (about 14 ounces each) vegetable broth
- 1 can (about 14 ounces) no-salt-added stewed tomatoes
- 8 ounces dried lentils, rinsed and sorted
- 2 teaspoons chili powder
- ½ teaspoon dried oregano
- 3 ounces uncooked whole wheat spaghetti, broken
- ¼ cup minced fresh cilantro

*Jalapeño peppers can sting and irritate the skin, so wear rubber gloves when handling peppers and do not touch your eyes.

1 Spray large nonstick saucepan with nonstick cooking spray; heat over medium heat. Add onions, carrot, celery, turnip and jalapeño pepper; cook and stir 10 minutes or until vegetables are crisp-tender.

2 Add water, broth, tomatoes, lentils, chili powder and oregano; bring to a boil. Reduce heat to low; cover and simmer 20 to 30 minutes or until lentils are tender.

3 Add pasta; cook 10 minutes or until tender. Ladle soup into bowls; sprinkle with cilantro.

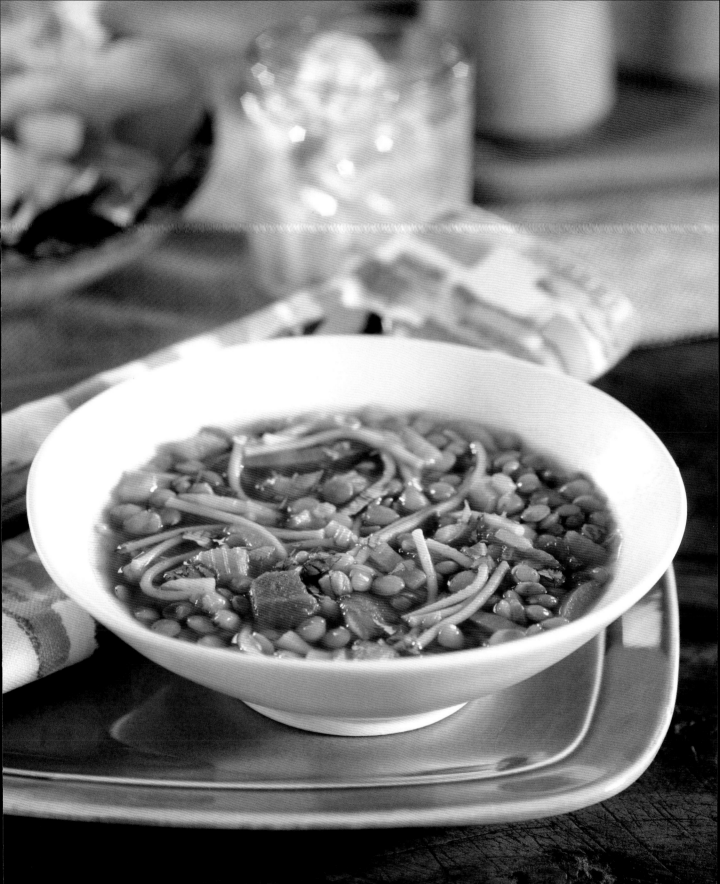

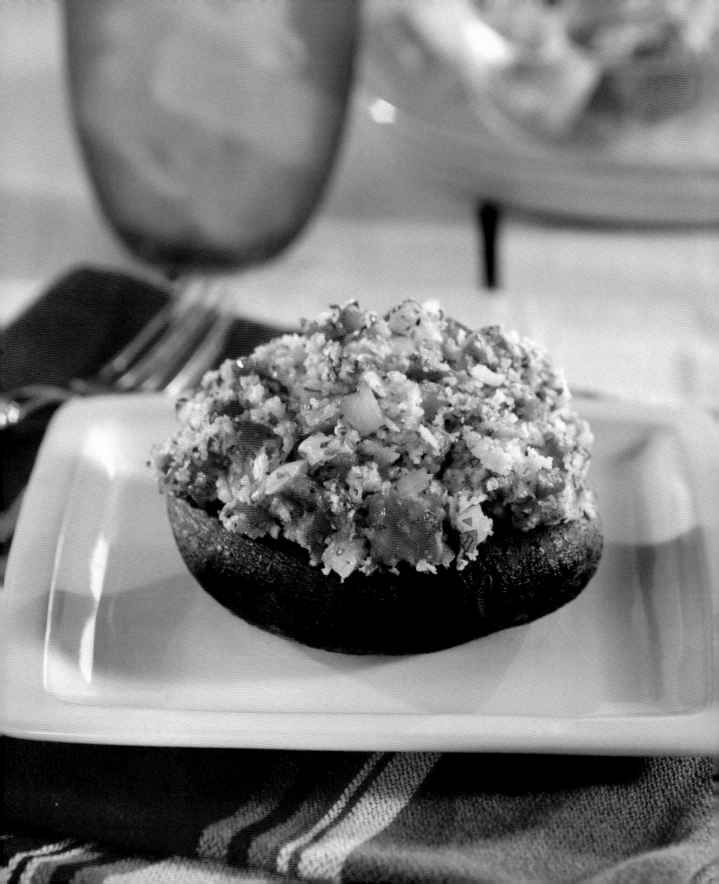

HEARTY SIDES

STUFFED PORTOBELLOS

  2 teaspoons olive oil

½ cup diced red bell pepper

½ cup diced onion

¼ teaspoon dried thyme

    Salt and black pepper

⅔ cup panko bread crumbs

⅔ cup diced fresh tomatoes *or* drained canned diced tomatoes

¼ cup grated Parmesan cheese

¼ cup chopped fresh parsley

  4 portobello mushroom caps

1 Preheat oven to 375°F.

2 Heat oil in medium nonstick skillet over medium-high heat. Add bell pepper and onion; cook and stir 5 minutes or until tender and lightly browned. Season with thyme, salt and black pepper.

3 Combine vegetable mixture, panko, tomatoes, Parmesan cheese and parsley in medium bowl. Place mushrooms, cap sides down, in shallow baking dish. Mound vegetable mixture on mushrooms. Bake 15 minutes or until mushrooms are tender and filling is golden brown.

BARLEY & VEGETABLE RISOTTO

MAKES 6 SERVINGS

4½ cups vegetable or chicken broth

2 teaspoons olive oil

1 small onion, diced

8 ounces sliced mushrooms

¾ cup uncooked pearl barley

1 large red bell pepper, diced

2 cups packed baby spinach

¼ cup grated Parmesan cheese

¼ teaspoon black pepper

1 Bring broth to a boil in medium saucepan. Reduce heat to low to keep broth hot.

2 Meanwhile, heat oil in large saucepan over medium heat. Add onion; cook and stir 4 minutes. Increase heat to medium-high. Add mushrooms; cook 5 minutes, stirring frequently, or until mushrooms begin to brown and liquid evaporates.

3 Add barley; cook 1 minute. Add broth, ¼ cup at a time, stirring constantly until broth is almost absorbed before adding the next. After 20 minutes of cooking, stir in bell pepper. Continue adding broth, ¼ cup at a time, until barley is tender (about 30 minutes total). Stir in spinach; cook and stir 1 minute or just until spinach is wilted. Stir in Parmesan cheese and black pepper.

Note

You may use your favorite mushrooms, such as button, crimini or shiitake, or a combination of two or more.

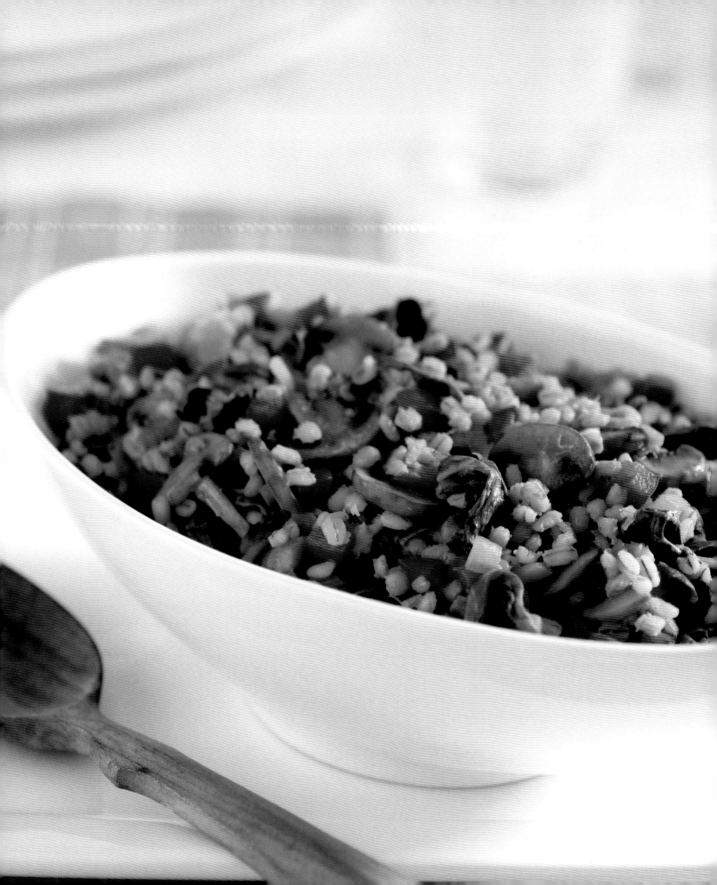

MIXED GRAIN TABBOULEH

MAKES 6 SERVINGS

1 cup uncooked long grain brown rice

3 cups canned chicken broth, divided

½ cup uncooked bulgur wheat

1 cup chopped tomatoes

½ cup minced green onions with tops

¼ cup fresh mint leaves, chopped

¼ cup fresh basil, chopped

¼ cup fresh oregano, chopped

3 tablespoons fresh lemon juice

3 tablespoons olive oil

½ teaspoon salt

½ teaspoon black pepper

1 Combine brown rice and 2 cups broth in medium saucepan. Bring to a boil over medium-high heat. Reduce heat to low. Simmer, covered, about 45 minutes or until broth is absorbed and rice is tender.

2 Combine bulgur and remaining 1 cup broth in small saucepan. Bring to a boil over medium-high heat. Reduce heat to low. Simmer, covered, 15 minutes or until broth is absorbed and bulgur is fluffy.

3 Combine tomatoes, green onions, chopped herbs, lemon juice, oil, salt and pepper in large bowl. Stir in rice and bulgur. Cool to room temperature.

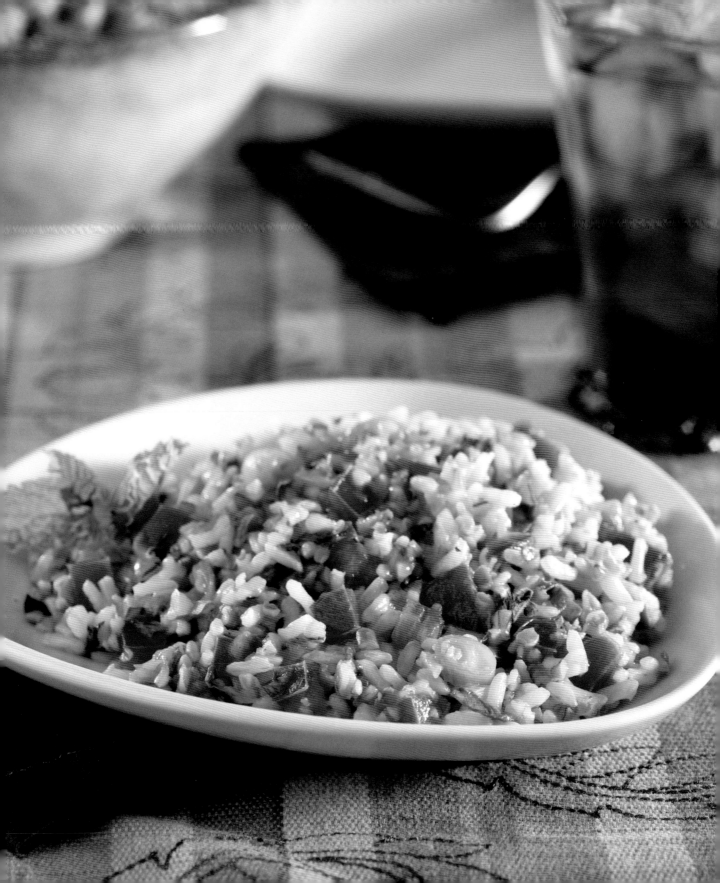

CORNMEAL-CRUSTED CAULIFLOWER STEAKS

MAKES 4 SERVINGS

½ cup cornmeal

¼ cup all-purpose flour

1 teaspoon salt

1 teaspoon dried sage

½ teaspoon garlic powder

Black pepper

½ cup milk

2 heads cauliflower

¼ cup (½ stick) butter, melted

Coleslaw and barbecue sauce (optional)

1 Preheat oven to 400°F. Line baking sheet with parchment paper.

2 Combine cornmeal, flour, salt, sage and garlic powder in shallow bowl or baking pan. Season with pepper. Pour milk into another shallow bowl.

3 Turn cauliflower stem side up on cutting board. Trim away leaves, leaving stem intact. Slice through stem into 3 slices. Trim off excess florets from end slices, creating flat "steaks." Repeat with remaining cauliflower. Reserve extra cauliflower for another use.

4 Dip cauliflower slices into milk to coat both sides. Place in cornmeal mixture; pat onto all sides of cauliflower. Place on prepared baking sheet; drizzle evenly with butter.

5 Bake 40 minutes or until cauliflower is tender. Serve with coleslaw on the side and barbecue sauce for dipping, if desired.

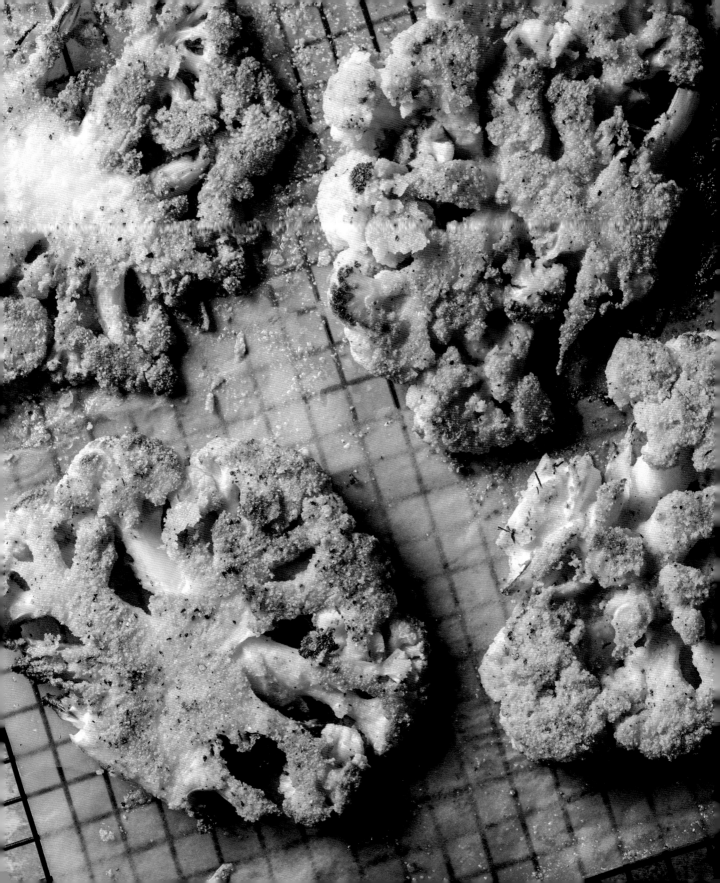

BUCKWHEAT WITH ZUCCHINI AND MUSHROOMS

MAKES 6 SERVINGS

1½ to 2 tablespoons olive oil

1 cup sliced mushrooms

1 medium zucchini, cut into ½-inch pieces

1 medium onion, chopped

1 clove garlic, minced

¾ cup buckwheat

¼ teaspoon dried thyme

¼ teaspoon salt

⅛ teaspoon black pepper

1¼ cups vegetable broth

Lemon wedges (optional)

1 Heat oil in large nonstick skillet over medium heat. Add mushrooms, zucchini, onion and garlic. Cook and stir 7 to 10 minutes or until vegetables are tender. Add buckwheat, thyme, salt and pepper; cook and stir 2 minutes.

2 Add broth; bring to a boil. Cover; reduce heat to low. Cook 10 to 13 minutes or until liquid is absorbed and buckwheat is tender. Remove from heat; let stand, covered, 5 minutes. Serve with lemon wedges, if desired.

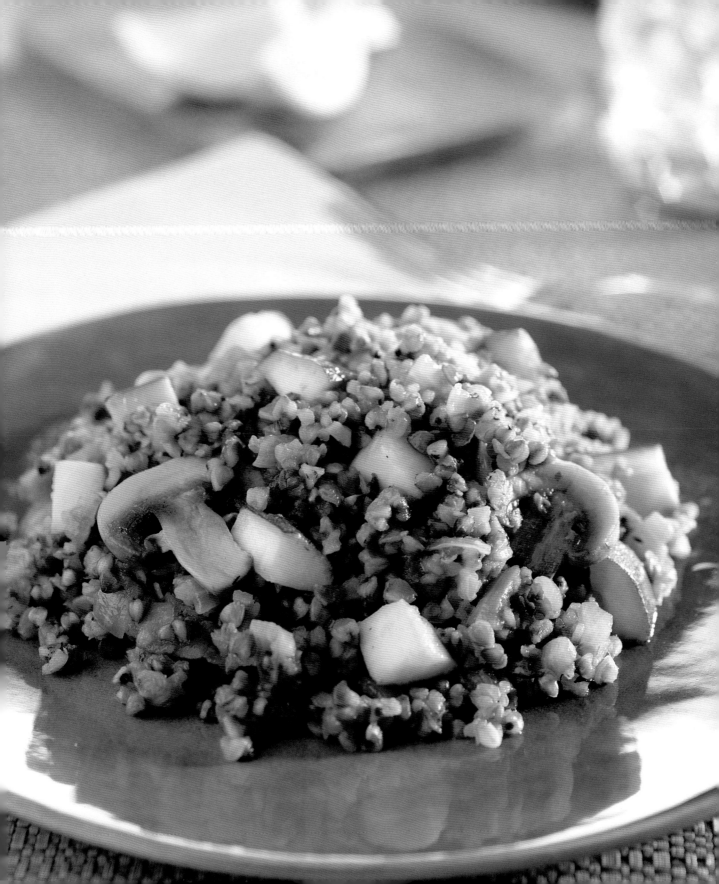

ASPARAGUS WITH RED ONION, BASIL AND ALMONDS

MAKES 4 SERVINGS

1 tablespoon olive oil

½ cup thinly sliced red onion, separated into rings

¼ cup vegetable broth

1 pound fresh asparagus, trimmed and cut into 1½-inch pieces

2 tablespoons chopped fresh basil

¼ teaspoon salt

¼ teaspoon black pepper

2 tablespoons sliced almonds, toasted*

*To toast almonds, place in nonstick skillet. Cook and stir over medium-low heat until nuts begin to brown, about 5 minutes. Remove immediately to plate to cool.

1 Heat oil in medium skillet over medium heat. Add onion; cover and cook 5 minutes or until wilted. Uncover; cook 4 to 5 minutes, stirring occasionally, until onion is tender and golden brown.

2 Bring broth to a boil in medium saucepan. Add asparagus; simmer over medium heat 3 minutes. Stir in onion; cook about 2 minutes or until asparagus is crisp-tender and most of liquid has evaporated. Stir in basil, salt and pepper. Transfer to serving plate. Sprinkle with almonds.

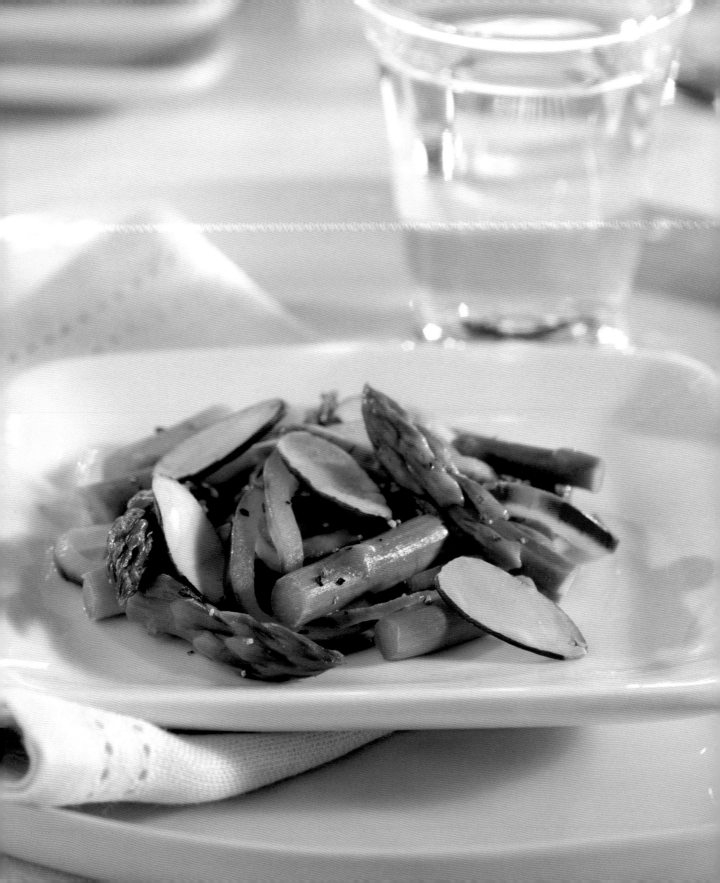

CONFETTI BLACK BEANS

MAKES 6 SERVINGS

1 cup dried black beans

1 can (about 14 ounces) vegetable broth

1 bay leaf

1 tablespoon olive oil

1 medium onion, chopped

¼ cup chopped red bell pepper

¼ cup chopped yellow bell pepper

2 cloves garlic, minced

1 jalapeño pepper,* finely chopped

1 large tomato, seeded and chopped

1 teaspoon salt

⅛ teaspoon black pepper

Hot pepper sauce (optional)

Jalapeño peppers can sting and irritate the skin, so wear rubber gloves when handling peppers and do not touch your eyes.

1 Sort and rinse beans; place in medium bowl. Cover with water. Soak 8 hours or overnight. Drain.

2 Combine beans and broth in large saucepan; bring to a boil over high heat. Add bay leaf. Reduce heat to low; cover and simmer 1½ hours or until beans are tender.

3 Heat oil in large nonstick skillet over medium heat. Add onion, bell peppers, garlic and jalapeño pepper; cook and stir 8 to 10 minutes or until onion is translucent. Add tomato, salt and black pepper; cook 5 minutes.

4 Add onion mixture to beans; cook 15 to 20 minutes.

5 Remove and discard bay leaf. Serve with hot pepper sauce, if desired.

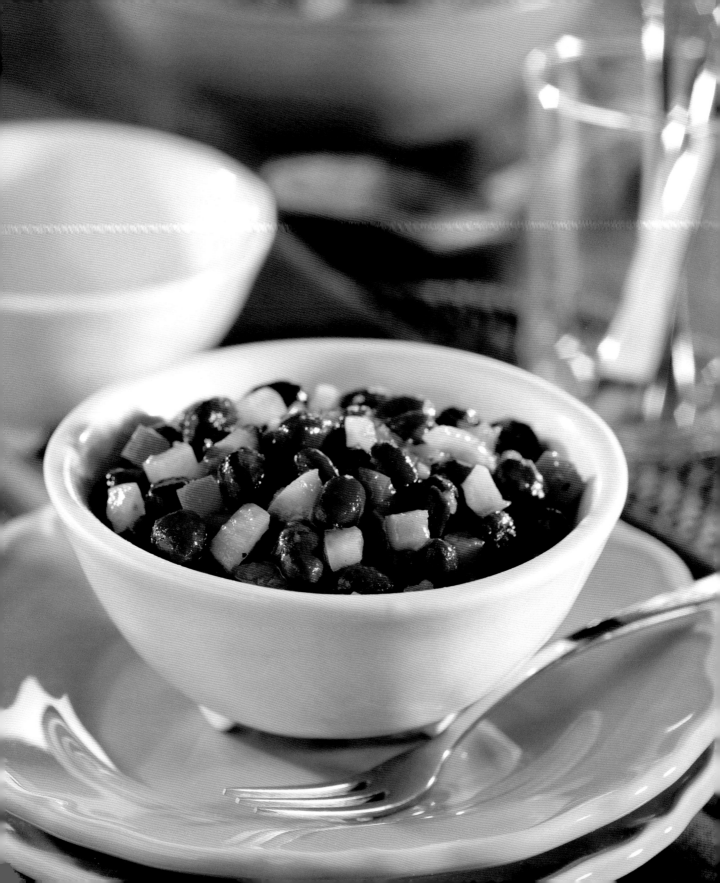

BROWN RICE WITH CHICKPEAS, SPINACH AND FETA

MAKES 4 SERVINGS

½ cup diced celery

½ cup uncooked instant brown rice

1 can (about 15 ounces) chickpeas, rinsed and drained

1 clove garlic, minced (optional)

1 package (10 ounces) frozen chopped spinach, thawed and squeezed dry

1 teaspoon Greek or Italian seasoning

¾ teaspoon vegetable broth

¼ teaspoon salt (optional)

⅛ teaspoon black pepper

2 cups water

1 tablespoon lemon juice

½ cup (2 ounces) crumbled feta cheese

1 Spray large skillet with nonstick cooking spray; heat over medium-high heat. Add celery; cook, stirring occasionally, 4 minutes or until lightly glazed and brown in spots.

2 Add rice, chickpeas, garlic, if desired, spinach, Greek seasoning, broth, salt, if desired, pepper and water. Stir to combine. Cover and bring to a gentle boil. Reduce heat to low and boil gently 12 minutes or until rice is tender. Remove from heat; add lemon juice and feta cheese. Mix gently with large spoon.

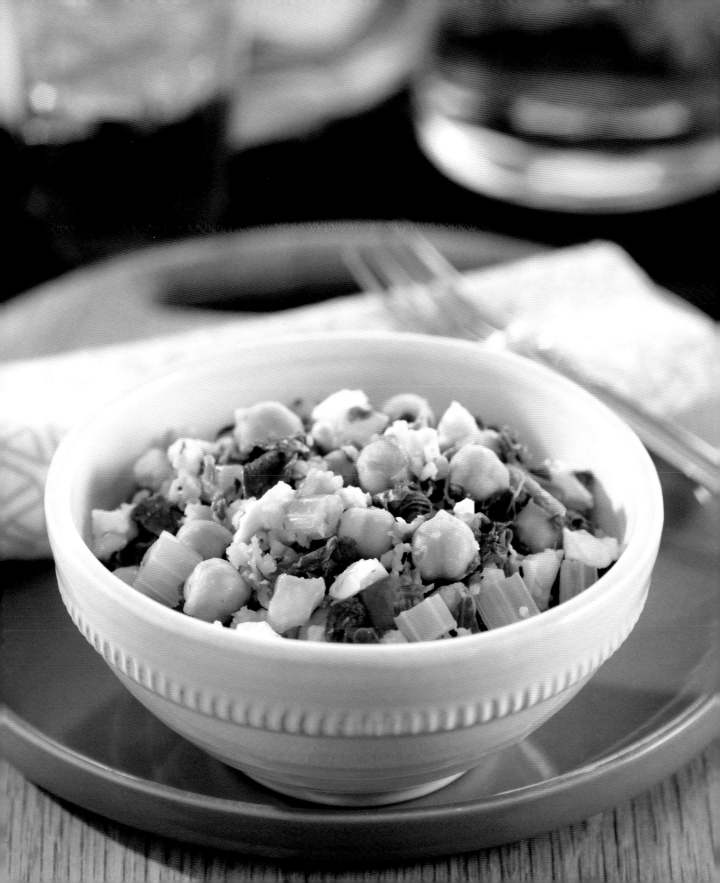

TIROKAFTERI (SPICY GREEK FETA SPREAD)

MAKES 2 CUPS

- 2 small hot red peppers
- ½ small clove garlic
- 1 block (8 ounces) feta cheese
- ¾ cup plain Greek yogurt
- 1 tablespoon lemon juice
- ½ teaspoon salt

  Toasted sliced French bread slices and/or cut-up fresh vegetables

1 Preheat oven to 400°F. Place peppers on small piece of foil on baking sheet. Bake 15 minutes or until peppers are soft and charred. Cool completely. Scrape off skin with paring knife. Cut off top and remove seeds. Place peppers in food processor. Add garlic; pulse until finely chopped.

2 Add feta cheese, yogurt, lemon juice and salt; pulse until well blended but still chunky. Store in airtight jar in refrigerator up to 2 weeks. Serve with bread, vegetables or cooked meats.

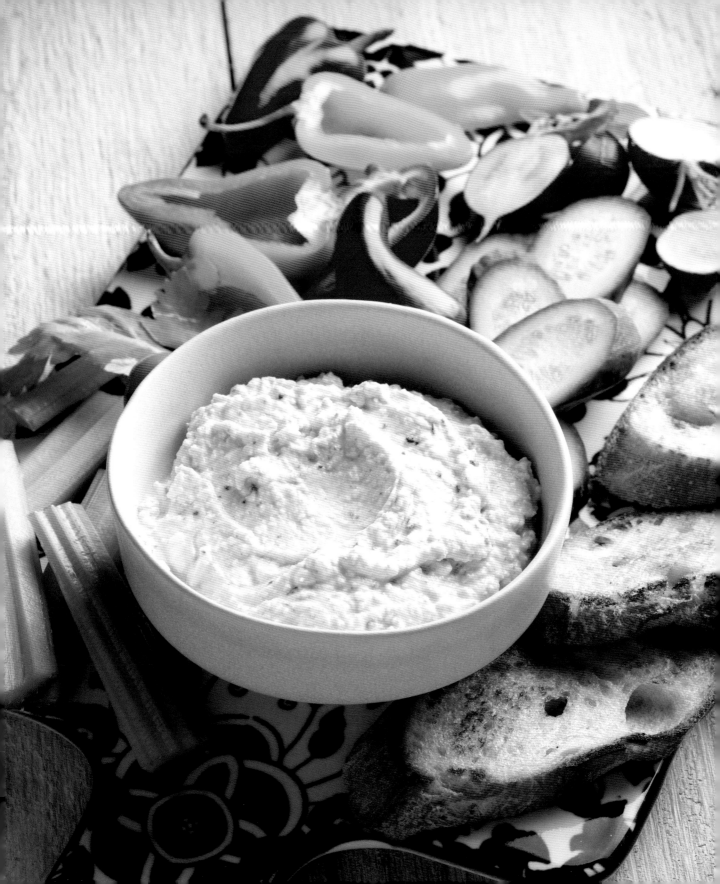

BULGUR PILAF WITH CARAMELIZED ONIONS & KALE

1 tablespoon olive oil

1 small onion, cut into thin wedges

1 clove garlic, minced

2 cups chopped kale

2 cups vegetable or chicken broth

¾ cup medium grain bulgur

½ teaspoon salt

¼ teaspoon black pepper

1 Heat oil in large nonstick skillet over medium heat. Add onion; cook about 8 minutes, stirring frequently or until softened and lightly browned. Add garlic; cook and stir 1 minute. Add kale; cook and stir about 1 minute or until kale is wilted.

2 Stir in broth, bulgur, salt and pepper. Bring to a boil. Reduce and simmer 12 minutes, covered, or until liquid is absorbed and bulgur is tender.

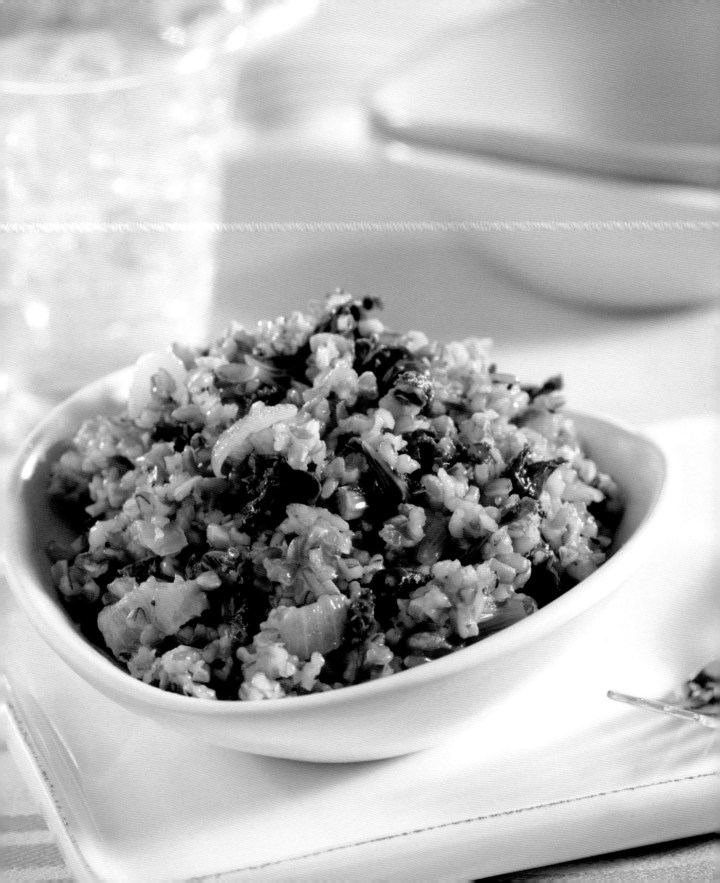

SPINACH-PINE NUT WHOLE GRAIN PILAF

MAKES 6 SERVINGS

2 cups hot cooked brown rice
  or bulgur

1½ ounces pine nuts or slivered
  almonds, toasted

2 ounces spinach leaves,
  coarsely chopped

1 tablespoon extra virgin
  olive oil

1 teaspoon dried basil

½ teaspoon salt

¼ teaspoon red pepper flakes

Place hot rice in large bowl. Add remaining ingredients and toss gently, yet thoroughly, until spinach is slightly wilted.

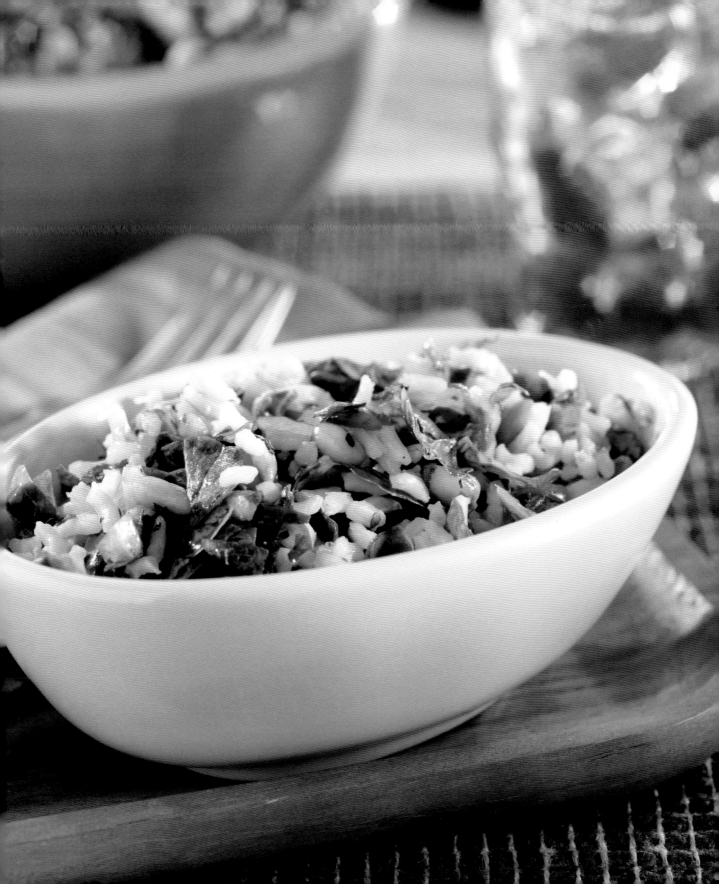

QUINOA TABBOULEH

MAKES 6 TO 8 SERVINGS

1 cup uncooked tricolor quinoa *or* ½ cup *each* red and white quinoa

2 cups water

2 teaspoons salt, divided

2 cups chopped fresh tomatoes (red, orange or a combination)

1 cucumber, quartered lengthwise and thinly sliced

¼ cup extra virgin olive oil

3 tablespoons fresh lemon juice

½ teaspoon black pepper

1 red or orange bell pepper, chopped

½ cup minced fresh parsley

1 Rinse quinoa in fine-mesh strainer under cold running water. Combine 2 cups water, quinoa and 1 teaspoon salt in medium saucepan. Bring to a boil over high heat. Reduce heat to low; cover and simmer 10 to 15 minutes until quinoa is tender and water is absorbed. Transfer to large bowl; cool to room temperature.

2 Meanwhile, combine tomatoes, cucumber and remaining 1 teaspoon salt in medium bowl. Let stand 20 minutes.

3 Stir cucumber, tomatoes and any accumulated juices into quinoa. Whisk oil, lemon juice and black pepper in small bowl until well blended. Stir into quinoa mixture. Add bell pepper and parsley; mix until well blended. Season with additional salt and pepper, if desired.

Note

For a heartier dish, add chickpeas. Drain 1 can (about 15 ounces) chickpeas, rinse under cold running water, and stir into quinoa with bell pepper.

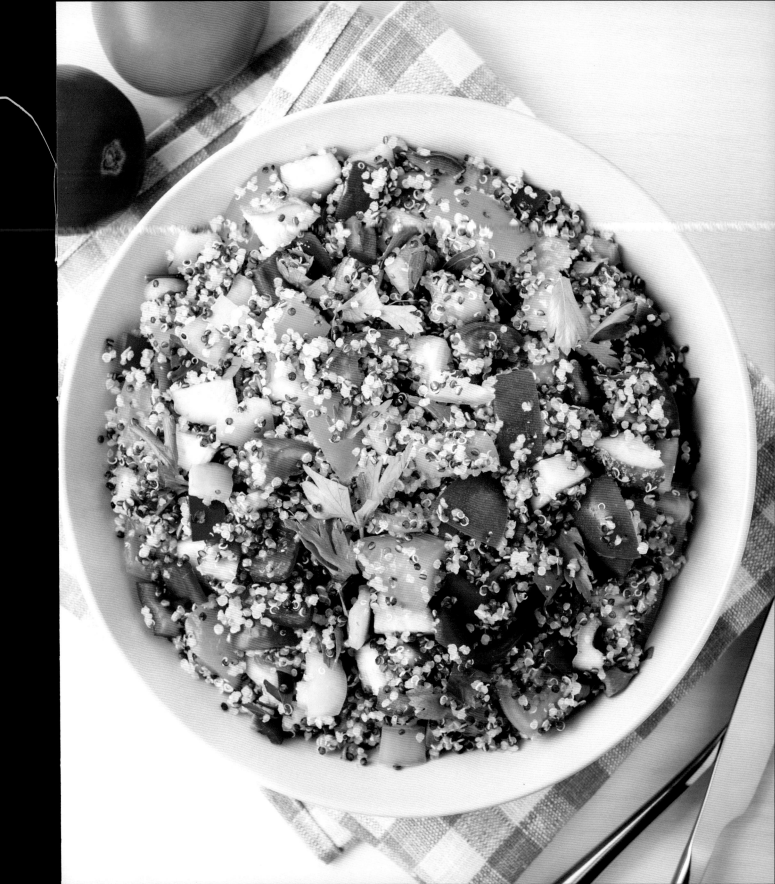

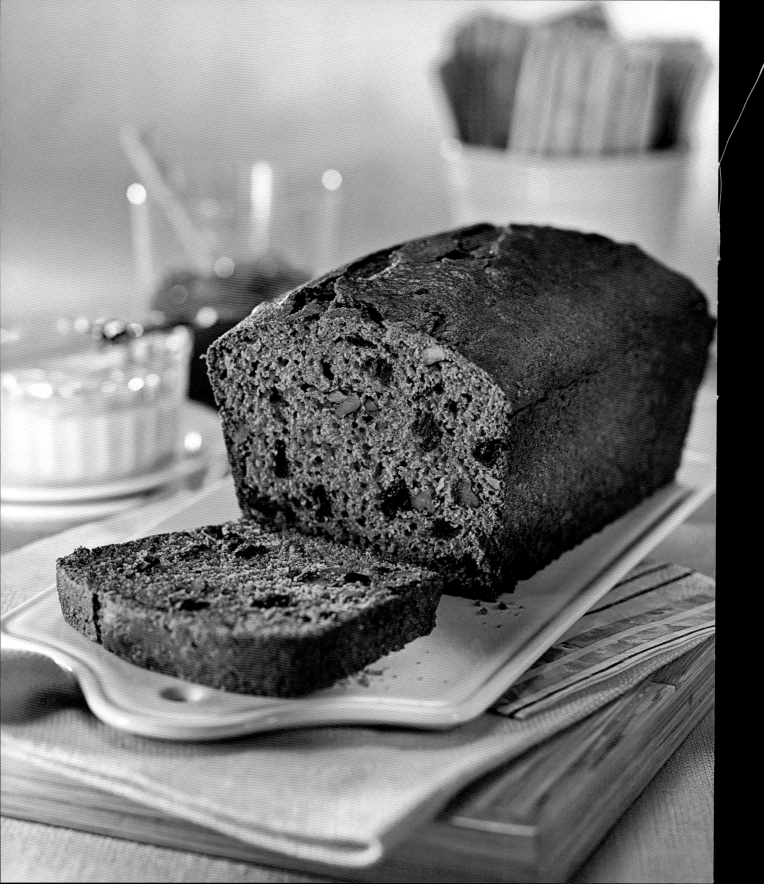

WHOLESOME BREADS & MUFFINS

HARVEST QUICK BREAD

- 1 cup all-purpose flour
- 1 cup whole wheat flour
- ½ cup packed brown sugar
- ¼ cup granulated sugar
- 1½ teaspoons baking powder
- ½ teaspoon baking soda
- ½ teaspoon ground cinnamon
- ½ teaspoon salt
- 1 egg
- 1 cup milk
- ¼ cup (½ stick) butter, melted
- ¾ cup dried cranberries
- ½ cup chopped walnuts

1 Preheat oven to 350°F. Spray 9×5-inch loaf pan with nonstick cooking spray.

2 Combine flours, sugars, baking powder, baking soda, cinnamon and salt in medium bowl; mix well. Whisk egg in large bowl. Stir in milk and butter; mix well. Gradually add flour mixture; stir just until dry ingredients are moistened. Stir in cranberries and walnuts just until combined. Pour batter into prepared pan.

3 Bake 45 to 50 minutes or until toothpick inserted into center comes out clean. Cool in pan 10 minutes; remove to wire rack to cool completely.

CRUNCHY WHOLE GRAIN BREAD

MAKES 2 LOAVES

2 cups warm water (105° to 115°F), divided

⅓ cup honey

2 tablespoons vegetable oil

1 tablespoon salt

2 packages (¼ ounce each) active dry yeast

2 to 2½ cups whole wheat flour, divided

1 cup bread flour

1¼ cups quick oats, divided

½ cup hulled pumpkin seeds or sunflower kernels

½ cup assorted grains and seeds

1 egg white

1 tablespoon water

1 Combine 1½ cups warm water, honey, oil and salt in small saucepan; heat over low heat until warm (115° to 120°F), stirring occasionally.

2 Dissolve yeast in remaining ½ cup warm water in large bowl of stand mixer; let stand 5 minutes. Stir in honey mixture. Add 1 cup whole wheat flour and bread flour; mix with dough hook at low speed 2 minutes. Slowly add 1 cup oats, pumpkin seeds and assorted grains; mix until incorporated. Add remaining whole wheat flour, ½ cup at a time; mix until dough begins to form a ball. Mix 6 to 8 minutes or until dough is smooth and elastic.

3 Place dough in greased bowl; turn to grease top. Cover and let rise in warm place 1½ to 2 hours or until doubled in size.

4 Spray two 9×5-inch loaf pans with nonstick cooking spray. Punch down dough. Divide dough in half; shape each half into a loaf. Place in prepared pans. Cover and let rise in warm place 1 hour or until almost doubled in size.

5 Preheat oven to 375°F. Beat egg white and 1 tablespoon water in small bowl. Brush over tops of loaves; sprinkle with remaining ¼ cup oats.

6 Bake 35 to 45 minutes or until breads sound hollow when tapped. Cool in pans 10 minutes; remove to wire racks to cool completely.

Tip

This bread makes a delicious and healthy way to use up various grains and seeds you may have on hand.

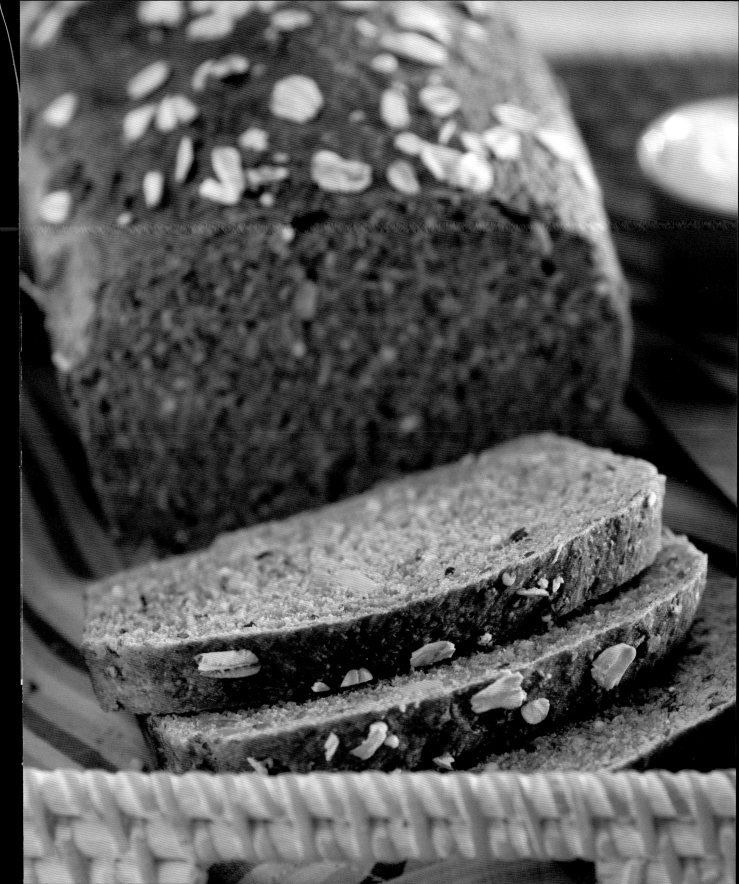

WHOLE-GRAIN
BANANA BREAD

¼ cup plus 2 tablespoons
    wheat germ, divided

⅔ cup butter, softened

1 cup sugar

2 eggs

1 cup mashed bananas
    (2 to 3 bananas)

1 teaspoon vanilla

1 cup all-purpose flour

1 cup whole wheat pastry
    flour

1 teaspoon baking soda

½ teaspoon salt

½ cup chopped walnuts or
    pecans (optional)

Slow Cooker Directions

1 Spray 1-quart casserole, soufflé dish or other high-sided baking pan with nonstick cooking spray. Sprinkle dish with 2 tablespoons wheat germ.

2 Beat butter and sugar in large bowl with electric mixer at medium speed until fluffy. Add eggs, one at a time; beat until blended. Add bananas and vanilla; beat until smooth.

3 Gradually stir in flours, remaining ¼ cup wheat germ, baking soda and salt. Stir in nuts, if desired. Pour batter into prepared dish; place in slow cooker. Cover; cook on HIGH 2 to 3 hours or until edges begin to brown and toothpick inserted into center comes out clean.

4 Remove dish from slow cooker. Cool on wire rack about 10 minutes. Remove bread from dish; cool completely on wire rack.

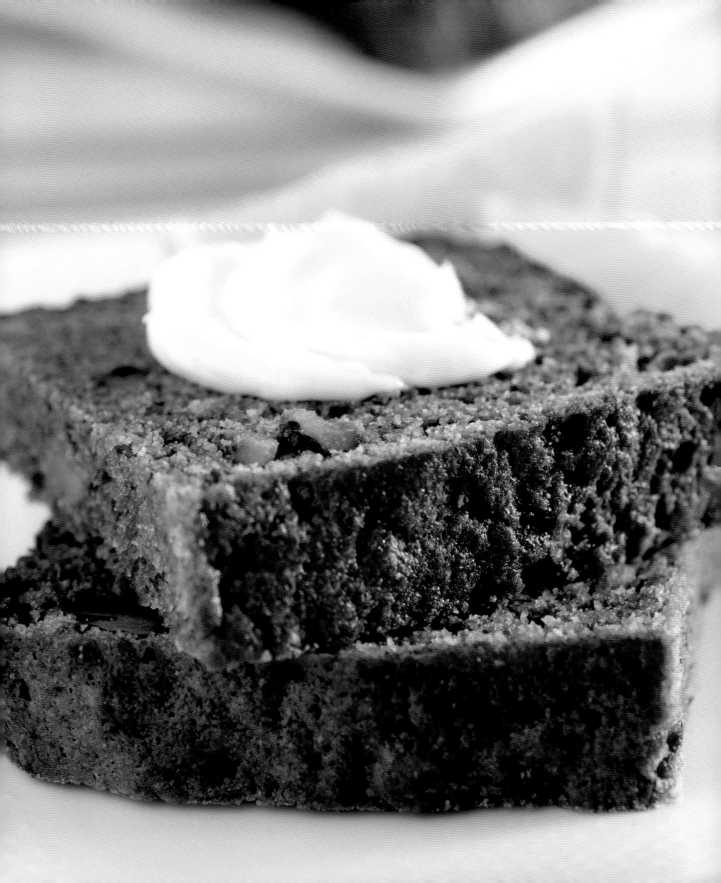

CARROT-PECAN MUFFINS

MAKES 18 MUFFINS

1 cup all-purpose flour

1 cup whole wheat flour

2 teaspoons baking powder

2 teaspoons ground cinnamon

1 teaspoon baking soda

¼ teaspoon salt

⅛ teaspoon ground cloves

2 eggs, lightly beaten

1 cup packed brown sugar

½ cup fat-free (skim) milk

¼ cup canola oil

¼ cup natural or unsweetened applesauce

1 teaspoon vanilla

2 cups finely shredded carrots

⅓ cup chopped pecans

1 Preheat oven to 375°F. Line 18 standard (2½-inch) muffin cups with paper baking cups or spray with nonstick cooking spray.

2 Combine flours, baking powder, cinnamon, baking soda, salt and cloves in large bowl; mix well. Whisk eggs and brown sugar in medium bowl until combined. Stir in milk, oil, applesauce and vanilla until smooth. Stir into flour mixture until combined. Fold in carrots and pecans. Spoon mixture evenly into prepared muffin cups.

3 Bake 18 to 20 minutes or until toothpick inserted into centers comes out clean. Cool in pans 5 minutes. Remove to wire racks; cool completely.

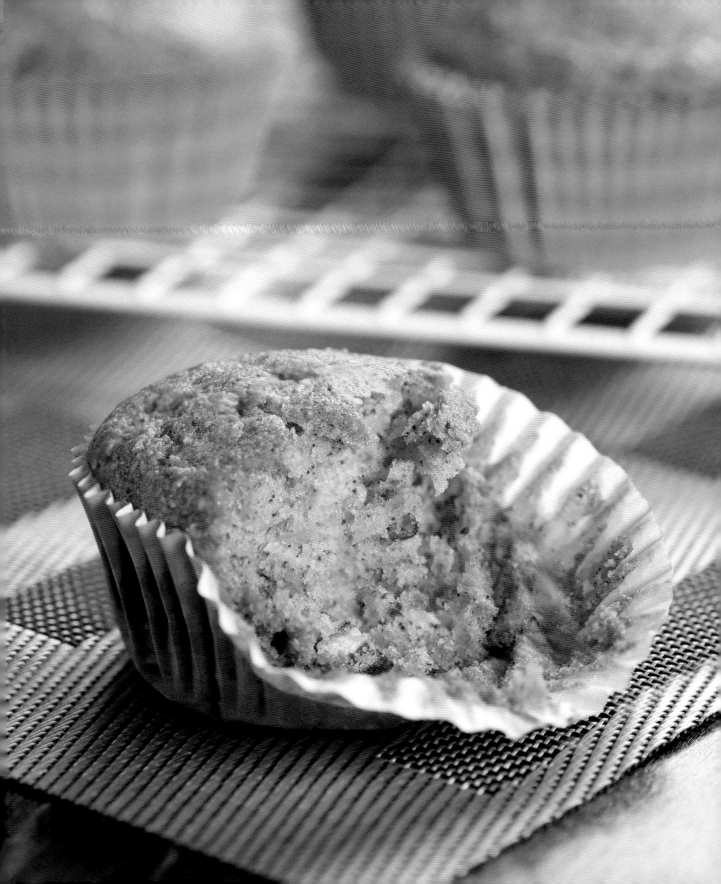

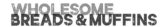

ZUCCHINI-DATE BREAD

Bread

- 1 cup chopped pitted dates
- 1 cup water
- 1 cup whole wheat flour
- 1 cup all-purpose flour
- 2 tablespoons granulated sugar
- 1 teaspoon baking powder
- ½ teaspoon baking soda
- ½ teaspoon salt
- ½ teaspoon ground cinnamon
- ¼ teaspoon ground cloves
- 2 eggs
- 1 small zucchini, finely chopped

Cream Cheese Spread (optional)

- 1 package (8 ounces) cream cheese
- ¼ cup powdered sugar
- 1 tablespoon vanilla
- ⅛ teaspoon ground cinnamon
   Dash ground cloves

1 Preheat oven to 350°F. Spray 8×4-inch loaf pan with nonstick cooking spray.

2 Combine dates and water in small saucepan; bring to a boil over medium-high heat. Remove from heat; let stand 15 minutes.

3 Combine flours, granulated sugar, baking powder, baking soda, salt, ½ teaspoon cinnamon and ¼ teaspoon cloves in large bowl. Beat eggs in medium bowl; stir in date mixture and zucchini. Stir egg mixture into flour mixture just until moistened. Pour into prepared pan.

4 Bake 30 to 35 minutes or until toothpick inserted into center comes out clean. Cool 5 minutes. Remove to wire rack; cool completely.

5 Meanwhile, prepare cream cheese spread, if desired. Beat cream cheese, powdered sugar, vanilla, ⅛ teaspoon cinnamon and dash cloves in small bowl until smooth and well blended. Cover and refrigerate until ready to use.

6 Cut bread into 16 slices. Serve with cream cheese spread, if desired.

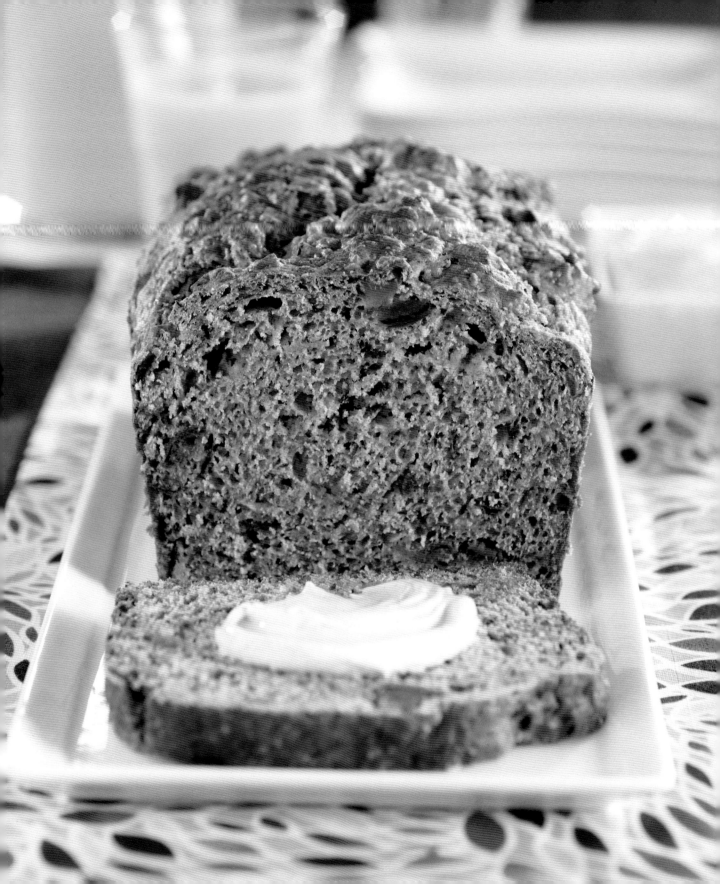

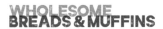

GOOD MORNING BREAD

1 cup mashed ripe bananas
  (about 3 medium)

¼ cup warm milk (130°F)

3 tablespoons vegetable or
  canola oil

2¼ cups bread flour, divided

¾ cup whole wheat flour

½ cup old-fashioned oats

1 package (¼ ounce) rapid-
  rise active dry yeast

1 teaspoon salt

1 teaspoon grated orange peel

1 teaspoon ground cinnamon

1 Combine bananas, milk and oil in medium bowl; mix well. Whisk ½ cup bread flour, whole wheat flour, oats, yeast, salt, orange peel and cinnamon in large bowl of electric stand mixer. Add banana mixture; beat at medium speed 3 minutes with paddle attachment.

2 Replace paddle attachment with dough hook; beat in enough remaining bread flour to form soft dough. Knead at medium-low speed 5 minutes or until dough is smooth and elastic. Place dough in greased bowl; turn dough so top is greased. Cover and let rise in warm place about 30 minutes or until doubled in size. (Dense loaf might not double in size.)

3 Spray 9×5-inch loaf pan with nonstick cooking spray. Punch down dough; shape into loaf. Place in prepared pan; cover and let rise in warm place about 30 minutes or until doubled in size. Preheat oven to 375°F.

4 Bake about 35 minutes or until browned and loaf sounds hollow when tapped and internal temperature reaches 200°F. Remove to wire rack to cool completely.

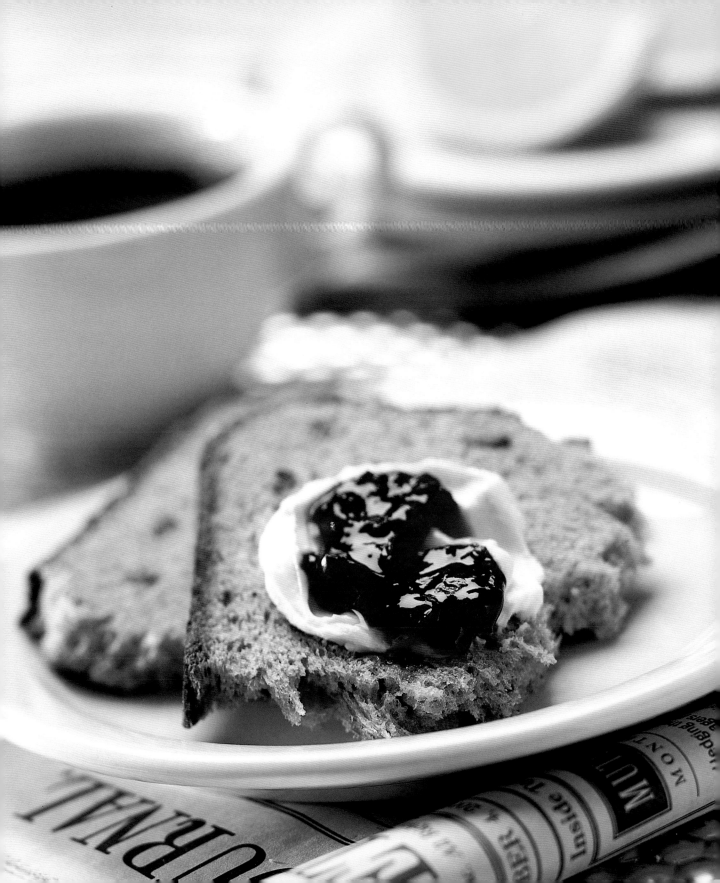

GINGER SQUASH MUFFINS

3 tablespoons water

1 tablespoon ground flaxseed

1½ cups all-purpose flour

⅓ cup whole wheat flour

⅓ cup granulated sugar

¼ cup packed dark brown sugar

2½ teaspoons baking powder

1 teaspoon ground cinnamon

½ teaspoon baking soda

¾ teaspoon salt

2 teaspoons ground ginger

1 cup frozen winter squash, thawed*

⅓ cup canola oil

¼ cup finely chopped walnuts

2 tablespoons finely chopped crystallized ginger (optional)

One 12-ounce package frozen squash yields about 1 cup squash. Or, use puréed cooked fresh butternut squash.

1 Preheat oven to 375°F. Grease 12 standard (2½-inch) muffin cups. Combine water and flaxseed in small saucepan; simmer over medium-low heat 5 minutes. Cool to room temperature.

2 Combine flours, sugars, baking powder, cinnamon, baking soda, salt and ground ginger in large bowl; mix well.

3 Combine squash, flaxseed mixture and oil in small bowl until well blended. Add to flour mixture; stir just until blended. *(Do not beat.)* Stir in walnuts and crystallized ginger, if desired. Spoon batter into prepared muffin cups, filling two-thirds full.

4 Bake 20 to 25 minutes or until toothpick inserted into centers comes out clean. Cool in pan 5 minutes. Remove to wire rack; cool completely.

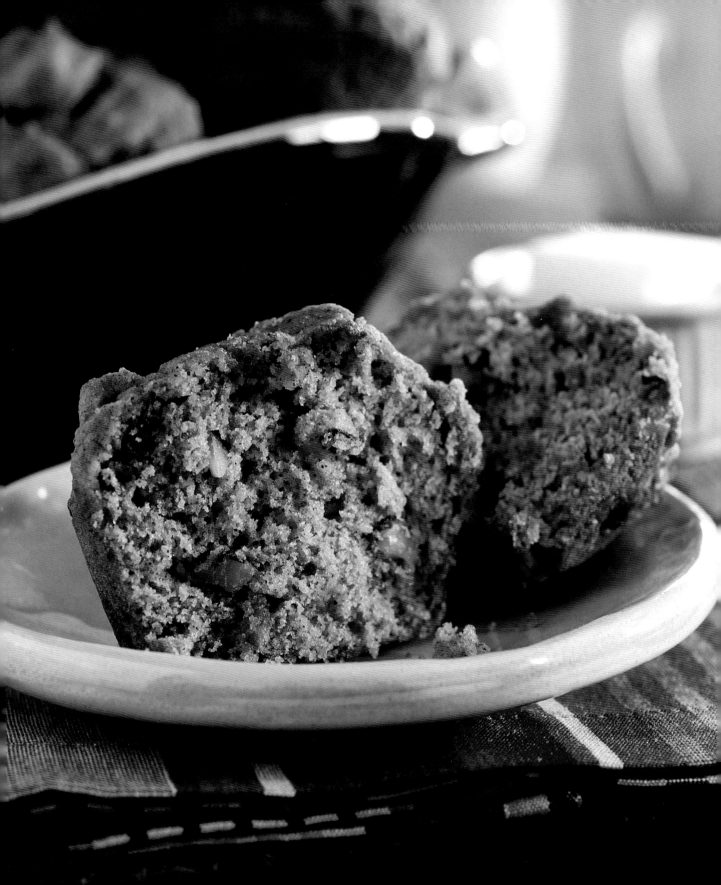

WHEAT GERM BREAD

- ¾ cup wheat germ, divided
- ¾ cup all-purpose flour
- ½ cup whole wheat flour
- ¼ cup packed light brown sugar
- 1 teaspoon baking soda
- ½ teaspoon baking powder
- ¼ teaspoon salt
- ½ cup raisins
- 1 cup buttermilk*
- ¼ cup (½ stick) margarine or butter, melted
- 1 egg

*You may substitute soured fresh milk. To sour milk, place 1 tablespoon lemon juice plus enough milk to equal 1 cup in 2-cup measure. Stir; let stand 5 minutes.

1 Preheat oven to 350°F. Spray 8×4-inch loaf pan with nonstick cooking spray. Measure 2 tablespoons wheat germ; set aside.

2 Combine remaining wheat germ, flours, brown sugar, baking soda, baking powder and salt in large bowl. Add raisins; stir until coated. Beat buttermilk, margarine and egg in small bowl until blended. Stir into flour mixture. Pour into prepared pan; sprinkle with reserved 2 tablespoons wheat germ.

3 Bake 40 to 50 minutes or until toothpick inserted into center comes out clean. Cool in pan on wire rack 10 minutes. Remove from pan and cool 30 minutes on wire rack.

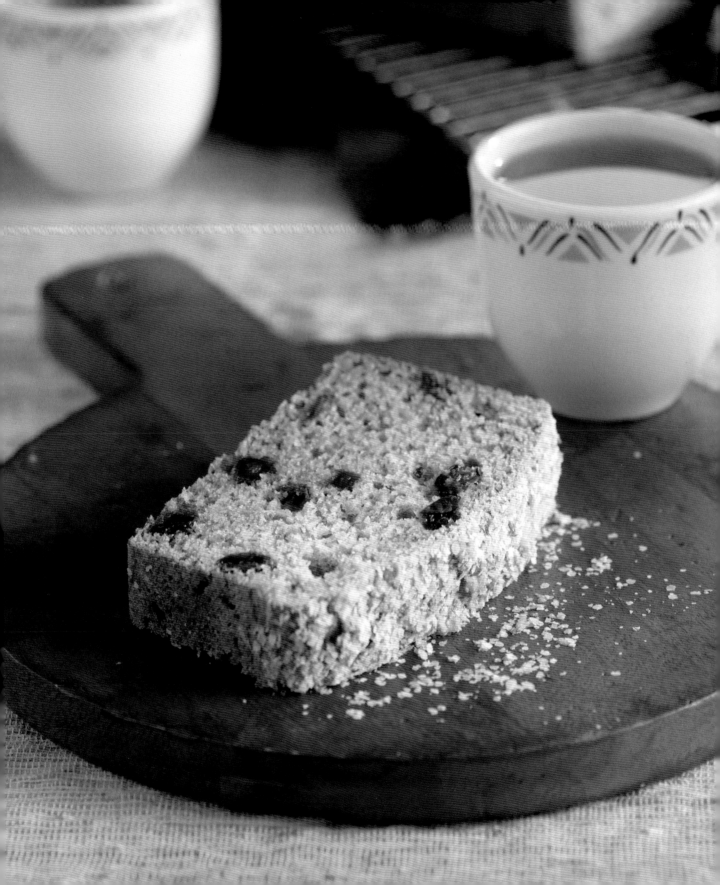

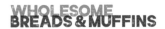

LEMON RAISIN QUICK BREAD

1¼ cups all-purpose flour

¾ cup whole wheat flour

4 tablespoons sugar, divided

2 teaspoons baking powder

½ teaspoon baking soda

¼ teaspoon salt

1½ cups lemon-flavored low-fat yogurt

¼ cup (½ stick) unsalted butter, melted and cooled slightly

1 egg

½ teaspoon grated lemon peel

1 cup raisins

¾ cup chopped walnuts (optional)

1 Preheat oven to 350°F. Grease 8×4-inch loaf pan.

2 Combine flours, 3 tablespoons sugar, baking powder, baking soda and salt in large bowl. Combine yogurt, butter, egg and lemon peel in medium bowl; stir until well blended. Pour yogurt mixture into flour mixture. Add raisins and walnuts, if desired; stir just until dry ingredients are moistened. Pour into prepared pan and smooth top. Sprinkle with remaining 1 tablespoon sugar.

3 Bake 40 to 45 minutes or until lightly browned and toothpick inserted into center comes out clean. Cool in pan on wire rack 30 minutes. Remove from pan; cool completely.

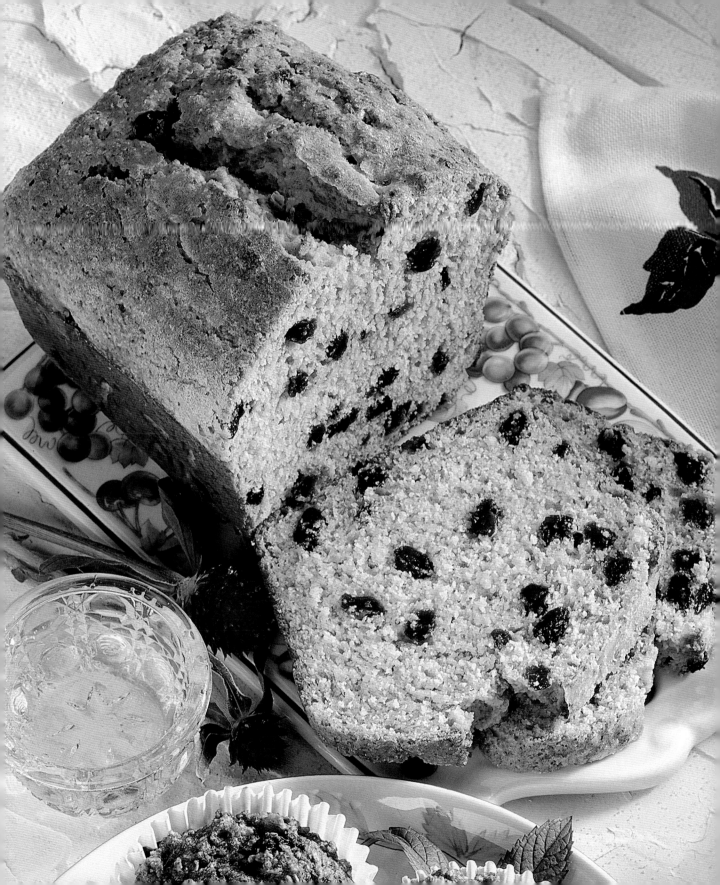

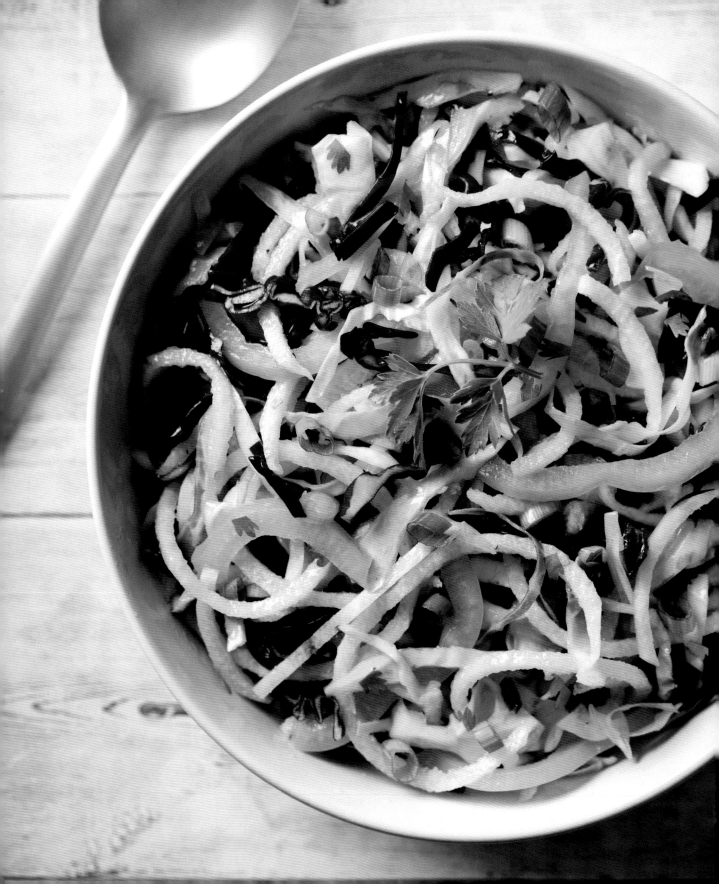

SATISFYING
SALADS & SLAWS

COLORFUL COLESLAW

¼ head green cabbage, shredded or thinly sliced

¼ head red cabbage, shredded or thinly sliced

1 small yellow or orange bell pepper, thinly sliced

1 small jicama, peeled and julienned

¼ cup thinly sliced green onions

2 tablespoons chopped fresh cilantro

¼ cup olive oil

¼ cup fresh lime juice

1 teaspoon salt

⅛ teaspoon black pepper

1 Combine cabbage, bell pepper, jicama, green onions and cilantro in large bowl.

2 Whisk oil, lime juice, salt and black pepper in small bowl until well blended. Pour over vegetables; toss to coat. Cover and refrigerate 2 to 6 hours for flavors to blend.

FATTOUSH SALAD

2 pita bread rounds

⅓ cup plus 3 tablespoons olive oil, divided

1 teaspoon salt, divided

2 cups chopped romaine or green leaf lettuce

1 seedless cucumber, quartered lengthwise and sliced

2 tomatoes, diced

4 green onions, thinly sliced

3 radishes, thinly sliced

¼ cup finely chopped fresh parsley

1 tablespoon finely chopped fresh mint

2 tablespoons pomegranate molasses

2 cloves garlic, minced

2 tablespoons red wine vinegar

1 tablespoon lemon juice

Black pepper

1 Preheat oven to 400°F. Cut pita bread rounds into 1-inch cubes. Toss with 3 tablespoons oil and ½ teaspoon salt in large bowl. Spread on large baking sheet. Bake 10 minutes or until pita cubes are browned and crisp. Cool completely on baking sheet.

2 Combine lettuce, cucumber, tomatoes, green onions, radishes, parsley and mint in large bowl. Add pita cubes.

3 For dressing, combine remaining ⅓ cup oil, molasses, garlic, vinegar and lemon juice in small bowl. Season with remaining ½ teaspoon salt and pepper; whisk until well blended. Taste and adjust seasoning. Pour over salad; toss until well blended and ingredients are coated.

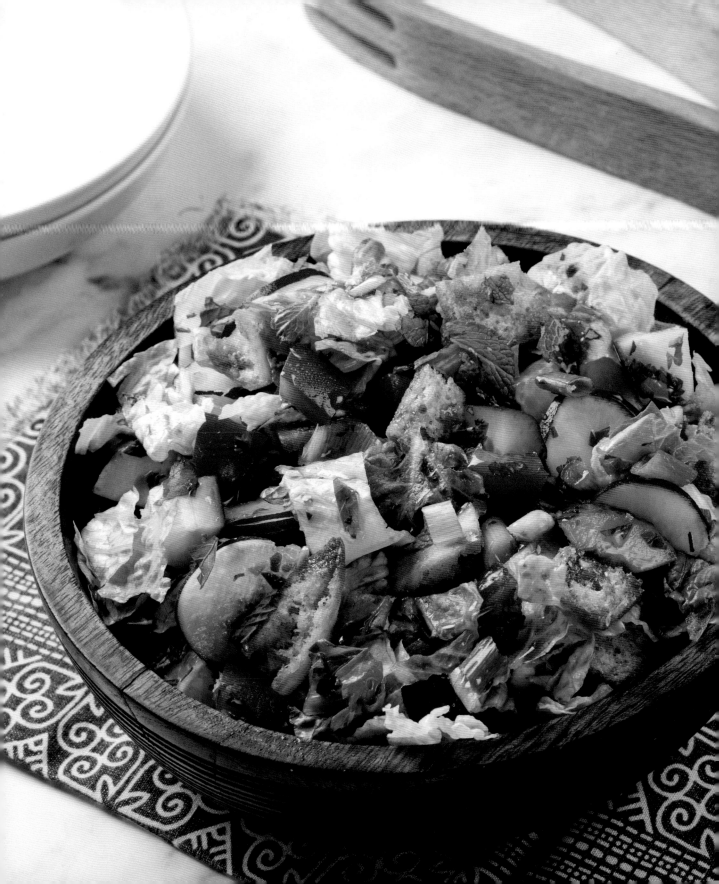

PINEAPPLE-GINGER SLAW WITH QUINOA

½ cup uncooked tricolored quinoa

1 cup water

¾ teaspoon salt, divided

4 cups shredded red cabbage

1 poblano pepper,* thinly sliced

½ cup chopped red onion

½ cup chopped fresh mint

3 tablespoons sugar

3 tablespoons fresh lime juice

2 tablespoons canola oil

2 teaspoons grated fresh ginger

1 can (8 ounces) pineapple tidbits, drained

Lime wedges (optional)

Poblano peppers can sting and irritate the skin, so wear rubber gloves when handling peppers and do not touch your eyes.

1 Rinse quinoa under cold running water in fine-mesh strainer. Bring 1 cup water, quinoa and ¼ teaspoon salt to a boil in small saucepan. Reduce heat to low; cover and simmer 10 to 15 minutes or until quinoa is tender and water is absorbed.

2 Place quinoa in fine-mesh strainer; rinse under cold running water to cool quickly.

3 Combine cabbage, poblano pepper, onion and mint in large bowl. For dressing, whisk sugar, lime juice, oil, ginger and remaining ½ teaspoon salt in small bowl.

4 Stir quinoa and pineapple into cabbage mixture. Add dressing; mix well. Serve with lime wedges, if desired.

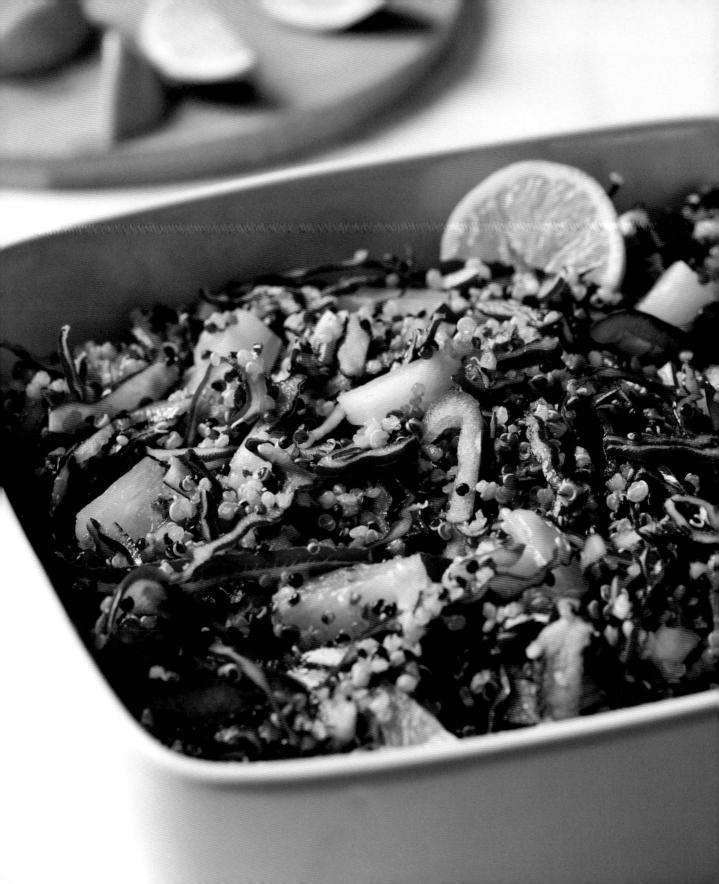

FARRO, CHICKPEA AND SPINACH SALAD

4 cups water

1 cup uncooked pearled farro

3 cups baby spinach, stemmed

1 medium cucumber, chopped

1 can (about 15 ounces) chickpeas, rinsed and drained

¾ cup pitted kalamata olives

¼ cup extra virgin olive oil

3 tablespoons white or golden balsamic vinegar *or* 3 tablespoons cider vinegar mixed with ½ teaspoon sugar

1 teaspoon chopped fresh rosemary

1 clove garlic, minced

1 teaspoon salt

⅛ to ¼ teaspoon red pepper flakes (optional)

½ cup (2 ounces) crumbled goat or feta cheese

1 Bring 4 cups water to a boil in medium saucepan. Add farro; reduce heat and simmer 20 to 25 minutes or until farro is tender. Drain and rinse under cold running water until cool.

2 Meanwhile, combine spinach, cucumber, chickpeas, olives, oil, vinegar, rosemary, garlic, salt and red pepper flakes, if desired, in large bowl. Stir in farro until well blended. Add goat cheese; stir gently.

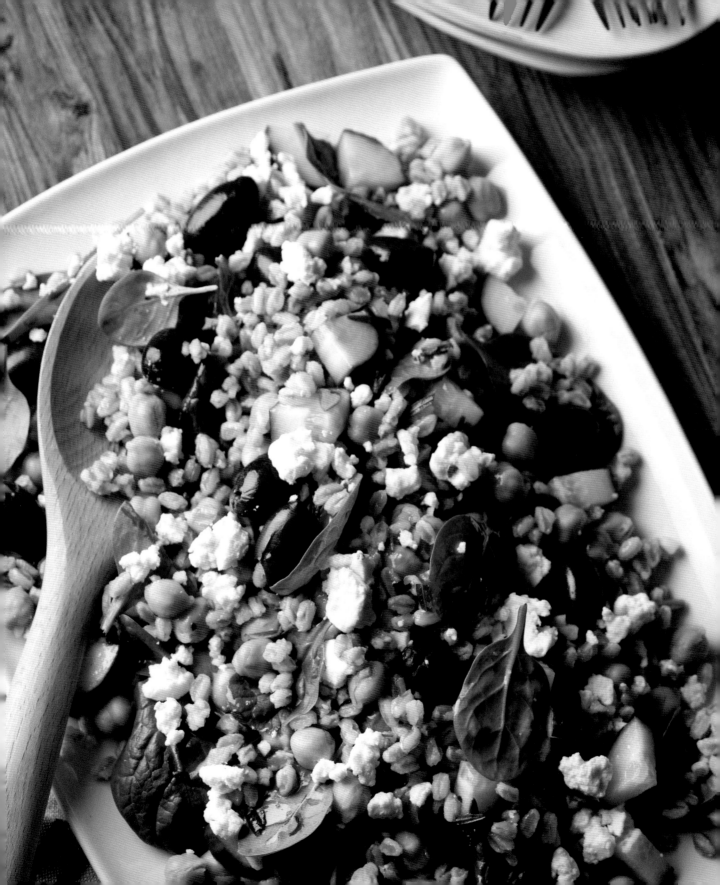

BEET AND ARUGULA SALAD

8 medium beets (5 to 6 ounces each)

⅓ cup red wine vinegar

¾ teaspoon salt

½ teaspoon black pepper

3 tablespoons extra virgin olive oil

1 package (5 ounces) baby arugula

1 package (4 ounces) crumbled goat cheese with garlic and herbs

1 Place beets in large saucepan; add water to cover by 2 inches. Bring to a boil over medium-high heat. Reduce heat to medium-low; cover and simmer 30 minutes or until beets can be easily pierced with tip of knife. Drain well; set aside until cool enough to handle.

2 Meanwhile, whisk vinegar, salt and pepper in large bowl. Slowly add oil in thin, steady stream, whisking until well blended. Remove 3 tablespoons dressing to medium bowl.

3 Peel beets and cut into wedges. Add warm beets to large bowl; toss to coat with dressing. Add arugula to medium bowl; toss gently to coat with dressing. Place arugula on platter or plates, top with beets and goat cheese.

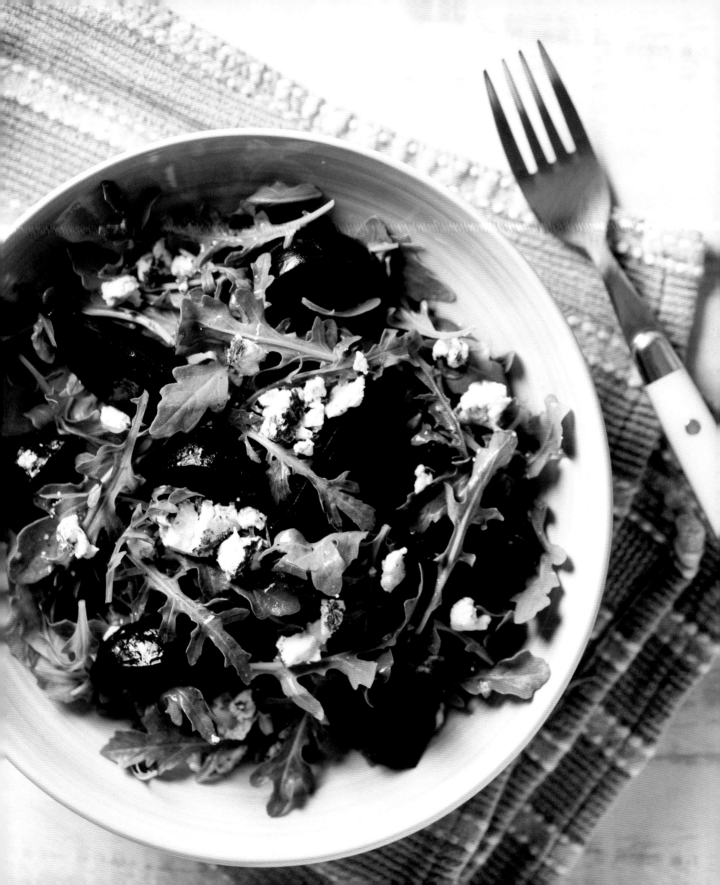

COLD PEANUT NOODLE AND EDAMAME SALAD

MAKES 4 SERVINGS

8 ounces uncooked whole wheat spaghetti

3 tablespoons reduced-sodium soy sauce

2 tablespoons unseasoned rice vinegar

2 tablespoons toasted sesame oil

1 tablespoon sugar

1 tablespoon finely grated fresh ginger

1 tablespoon creamy peanut butter

1 tablespoon sriracha or hot chili sauce

2 teaspoons minced garlic

½ cup thawed frozen shelled edamame

1 small seedless cucumber (8 ounces), thinly sliced

2 large carrots, slivered

¼ cup sliced green onions

¼ cup chopped peanuts

1 Cook noodles according to package directions. Rinse under cold running water; drain. Cut noodles into 3-inch lengths. Place in large bowl; set aside.

2 Whisk soy sauce, vinegar, oil, sugar, ginger, peanut butter, sriracha and garlic in small bowl until smooth and well blended.

3 Gently toss noodles with dressing. Stir in edamame, cucumber and carrots. Cover and refrigerate at least 30 minutes to allow flavors to blend.

4 Sprinkle with green onions and peanuts just before serving.

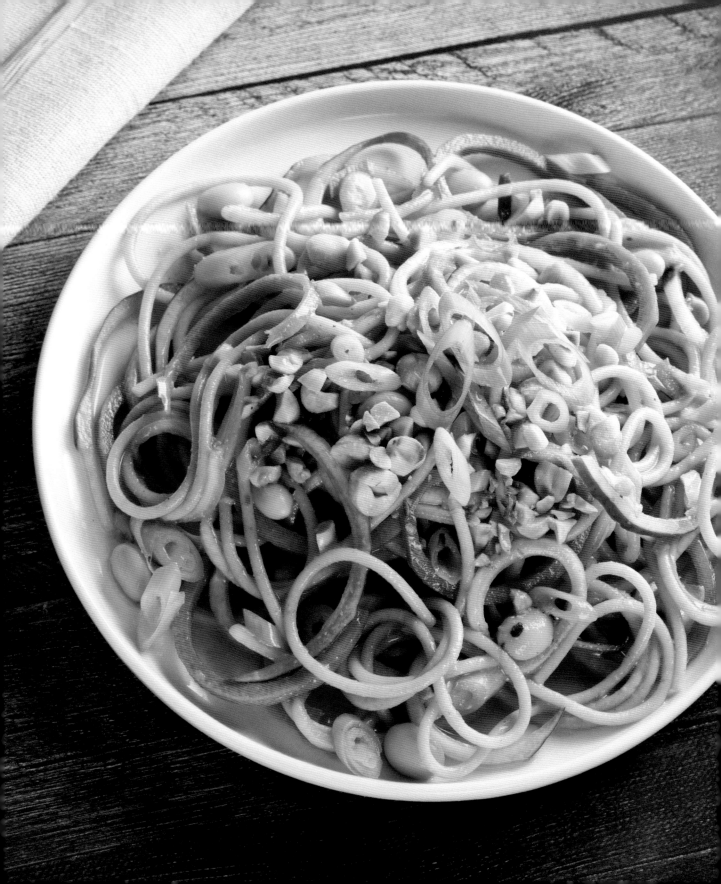

EDAMAME PEANUT SLAW

4 cups thinly sliced green cabbage

3 cups thinly sliced red cabbage (about ½ of a small head)

1 red bell pepper, thinly sliced

1 cup thawed frozen shelled edamame

3 green onions, thinly sliced

1 carrot, shredded or julienned

Juice of 1 lime

2 tablespoons unseasoned rice vinegar

1 tablespoon dark sesame oil

2 teaspoons salt

1 teaspoon sugar

1 teaspoon minced fresh ginger

1 cup roasted peanuts

Combine cabbage, bell pepper, edamame, green onions and carrot in large bowl. Whisk lime juice, vinegar, oil, salt, sugar and ginger in small bowl until salt and sugar are dissolved. Pour dressing over salad; mix well. Stir in peanuts just before serving.

Note

This can be made at least 1 day ahead of time, but will even be good for several days. Store in a covered bowl or container and adjust the salt, lime juice and vinegar before serving. For crunchy peanuts, stir them in just before serving. They will also be fine if you stir them in early and let them sit. Their texture will be more crisp-tender than crisp, similar to the edamame.

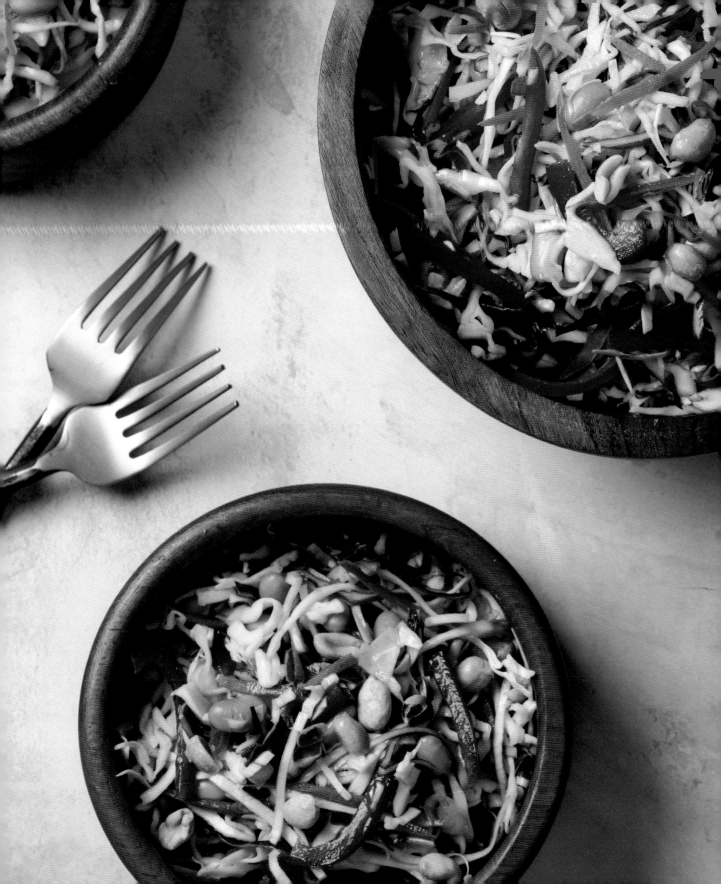

CAULIFLOWER CHOPPED SALAD

Cauliflower

- ½ cup red wine vinegar
- ¼ cup olive oil
- 1 teaspoon salt
- 1 teaspoon honey
- 1 teaspoon Dijon mustard
- ½ teaspoon dried oregano
- 1 clove garlic, minced
- ¼ teaspoon black pepper
- 2 cups small cauliflower florets (½ inch)

Salad

- 1 head iceberg lettuce, chopped
- 1 container (4 ounces) crumbled blue cheese
- 1 pint grape tomatoes, halved *or* 1 cup finely chopped tomatoes
- ½ cup finely chopped red onion
- 2 green onions, finely chopped
- 1 avocado, diced

1 For cauliflower, whisk vinegar, oil, salt, honey, mustard, oregano, garlic and pepper in medium bowl. Add cauliflower; stir to coat. Cover and refrigerate several hours or overnight.

2 For salad, combine lettuce, blue cheese, tomatoes, red onion and green onions in large bowl; toss to coat. Remove cauliflower from marinade using slotted spoon; place on salad. Whisk marinade; pour over salad and toss to coat. Top with avocado; mix gently.

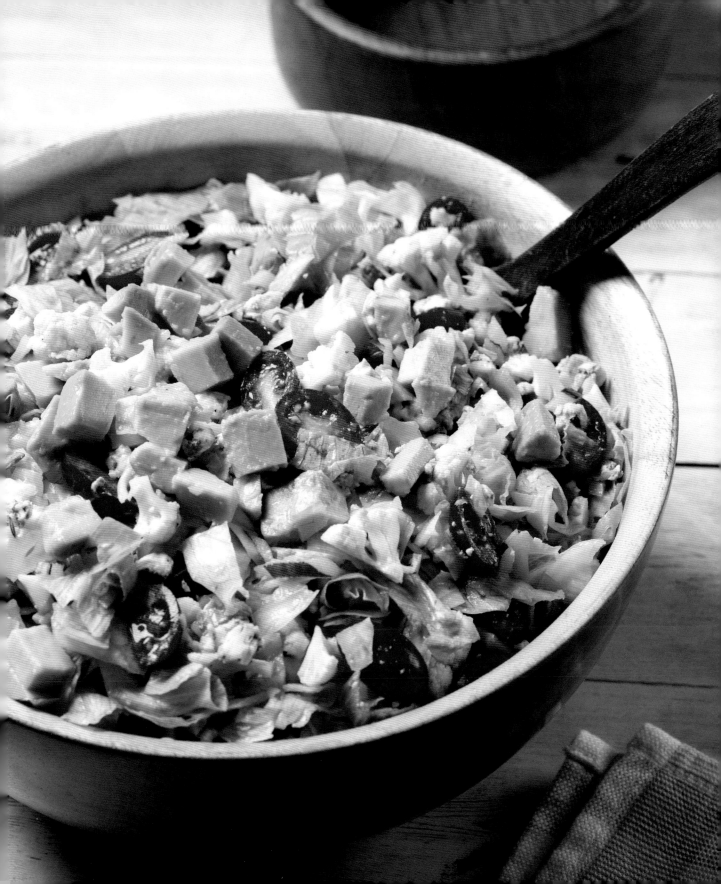

KALE SALAD WITH CHERRIES AND AVOCADOS

MAKES 6 TO 8 SERVINGS

¼ cup plus 1 teaspoon olive oil, divided

3 tablespoons uncooked quinoa

¾ teaspoon salt, divided

3 tablespoons balsamic vinegar

1 tablespoon red wine vinegar

1 tablespoon maple syrup

2 teaspoons Dijon mustard

¼ teaspoon dried oregano

⅛ teaspoon black pepper

1 large bunch kale (about 1 pound)

1 package (5 ounces) dried cherries

2 avocados, diced

½ cup smoked almonds, chopped

1 Heat 1 teaspoon oil in small saucepan over medium-high heat. Add quinoa; cook and stir 3 to 5 minutes or until quinoa is golden brown and popped. Season with ¼ teaspoon salt. Remove to plate; cool completely.

2 Combine balsamic vinegar, red wine vinegar, maple syrup, mustard, oregano, pepper and remaining ½ teaspoon salt in medium bowl. Whisk in remaining ¼ cup oil until well blended.

3 Place kale in large bowl. Pour dressing over kale; massage dressing into leaves until well blended and kale is slightly softened. Add popped quinoa; stir until well blended. Add cherries, avocados and almonds; toss until blended.

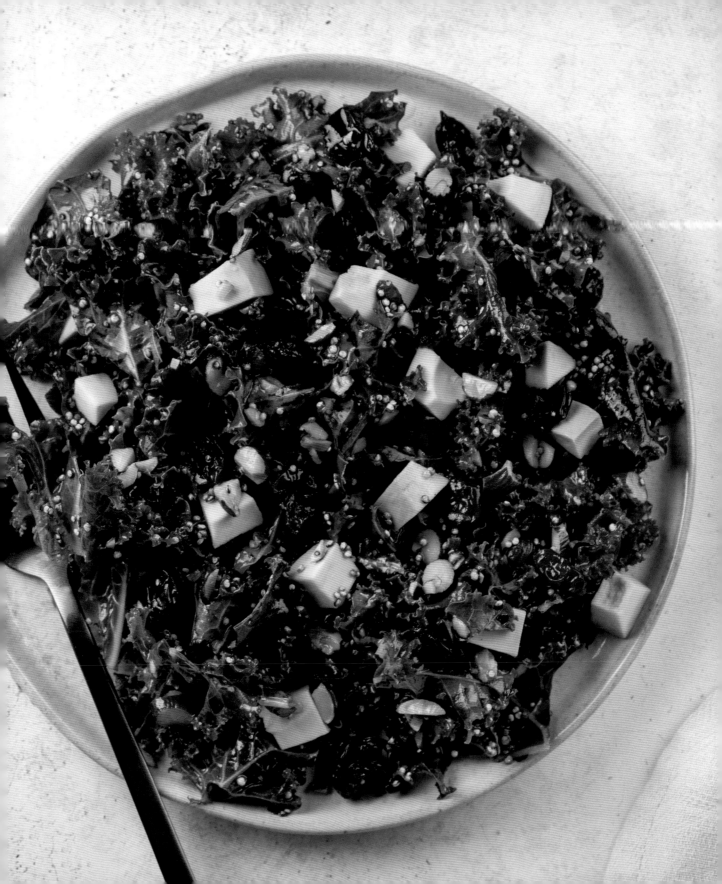

HOUSE SALAD

Dressing

½ cup mayonnaise

½ cup white wine vinegar

¼ cup grated Parmesan cheese

1 tablespoon olive oil

1 tablespoon lemon juice

1 tablespoon corn syrup

1 clove garlic, minced

¾ teaspoon Italian seasoning

½ teaspoon salt

½ teaspoon black pepper

Salad

1 package (10 ounces) Italian salad blend

2 plum tomatoes, thinly sliced

1 cup croutons or Homemade Croutons (see Note)

½ cup thinly sliced red or green bell pepper

½ cup thinly sliced red onion

¼ cup sliced black olives

   Pepperoncini peppers (optional)

1 Prepare Homemade Croutons, if desired.

2 For dressing, whisk mayonnaise, vinegar, Parmesan cheese, oil, lemon juice, corn syrup, garlic, Italian seasoning, salt and black pepper in medium bowl until well blended.

3 For salad, place salad blend in large bowl; top with tomatoes, croutons, bell pepper, onion, olives and pepperoncini, if desired. Add dressing; toss to coat.

Homemade Croutons

Homemade croutons are incredibly easy to make and much better than store-bought versions. They make a versatile topping for any salad, soup or even pasta dish and keep well in an airtight container at room temperature, so make extras to have on hand. Bonus—croutons are a great way to use up stale bread. If you have stale bread but aren't ready to make croutons, put it in a freezer bag and freeze it until you're ready. Preheat oven to 350°F. Cut any kind of bread into cubes. Hearty bread like whole wheat, Tuscan or sourdough works best, but sandwich bread works, too. Spread the bread on sheet pan and drizzle with olive oil. Toss with spatula or hands to coat. The bread should be evenly coated; add more oil if needed and toss again. If desired, season with salt and pepper and dried herbs like oregano, thyme or rosemary. Bake 10 to 15 minutes or until golden brown, stirring once or twice. Cool on sheet pan before serving.

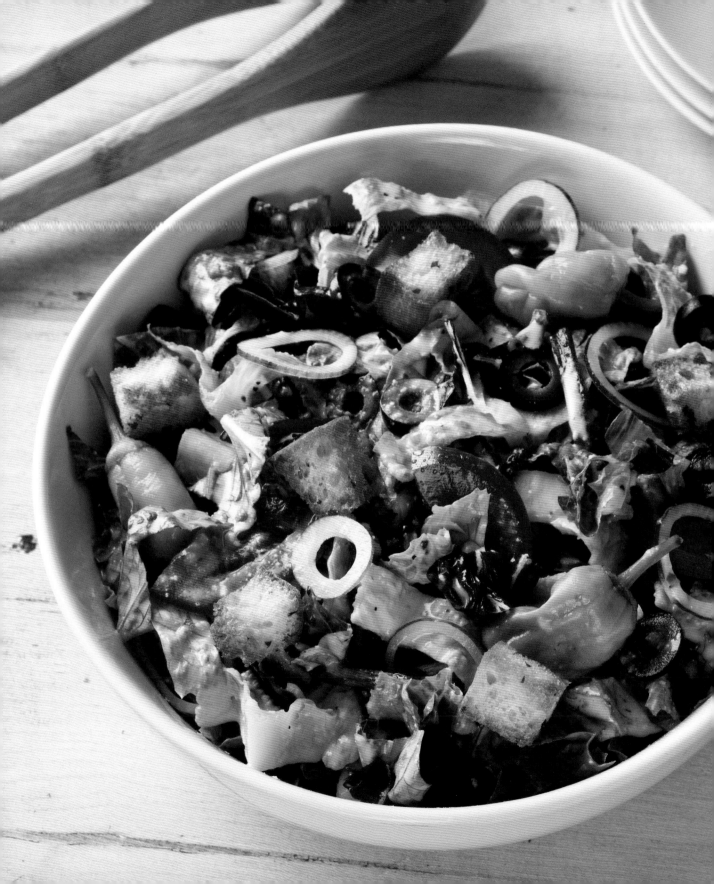

SHRIMP AND SOBA NOODLE SALAD

    4 ounces soba noodles

    2 cups diagonally sliced green
      beans (bite-size pieces)

1½ cups sliced mushrooms

1½ cups (6 ounces) cooked
      medium shrimp (with
      tails on)

    ¼ cup thinly sliced red bell
      pepper

    2 tablespoons orange juice

    2 tablespoons lime juice

    1 tablespoon reduced-sodium
      soy sauce

    2 teaspoons dark sesame oil

    2 tablespoons finely chopped
      fresh cilantro

    1 to 2 tablespoons toasted
      sesame seeds (optional)

1 Cook noodles according to package directions omitting any salt or fat. Drain, rinse under warm water. Drain again and transfer to large bowl.

2 Spray large skillet with nonstick cooking spray; heat over medium-high heat. Add green beans and mushrooms; cook, mixing occasionally, 8 minutes or until mushrooms are lightly browned and beans are softened.

3 Combine noodles, shrimp, green bean mixture and bell pepper in large bowl. Whisk orange juice, lime juice, soy sauce and oil in small bowl. Pour over salad, sprinkle with cilantro and sesame seeds, if desired. Toss gently.

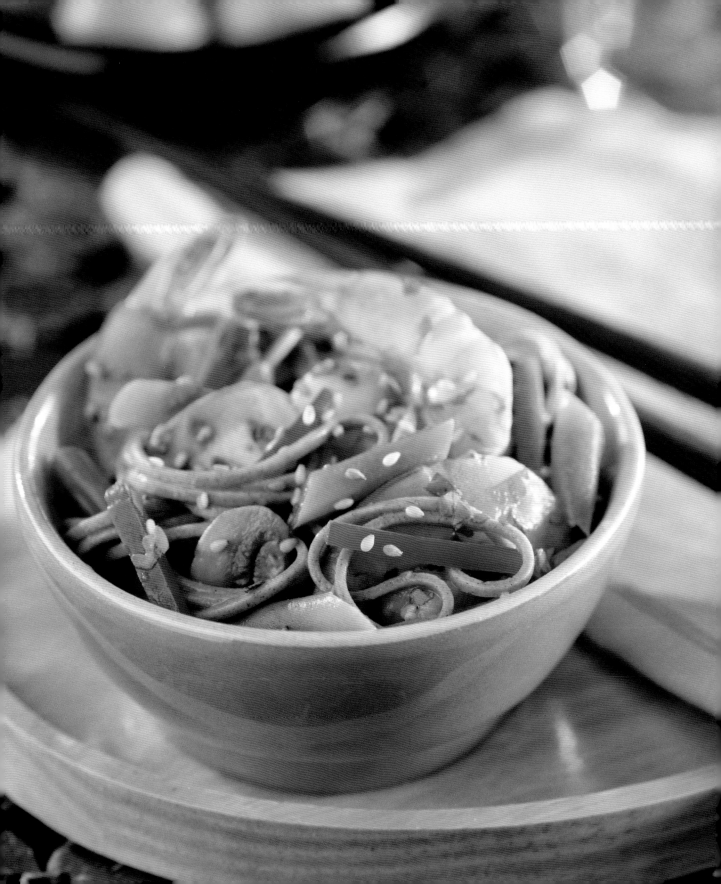

QUINOA AND CAULIFLOWER TACO SALAD

¾ cup uncooked quinoa

1½ cups water

4 cloves garlic, minced, divided

1 tablespoon chili powder

1¾ teaspoons salt, divided

1¼ teaspoons ground cumin, divided

½ teaspoon dried oregano

¼ cup plus 2 teaspoons olive oil, divided

4 cups coarsely chopped cauliflower

½ cup pepitas (pumpkin seeds)

Juice of 1 lime

Salt and black pepper

4 to 6 cups shredded iceberg lettuce

2 tomatoes, diced

2 avocados, diced

Shredded Cheddar cheese or crumbled cotija cheese

Crispy tortilla strips or crushed tortilla chips

1 Rinse quinoa in fine-mesh strainer under cold water. Place in medium saucepan. Add 1½ cups water, 3 cloves garlic, chili powder, 1 teaspoon salt, 1 teaspoon cumin and oregano. Bring to a boil over medium-high heat. Reduce heat to low; cover and simmer 15 minutes or until quinoa is tender and most of water is absorbed.

2 Meanwhile, heat 1 teaspoon oil in large nonstick skillet over medium-high heat. Add cauliflower and ½ teaspoon salt; cook and stir 10 minutes or until tender and browned. Add quinoa to cauliflower; cook and stir until well blended.

3 Heat 1 teaspoon oil in small skillet over medium heat. Add pepitas; cook and stir 3 to 5 minutes or until they begin to pop and are lightly browned. Remove from heat. Season with remaining ¼ teaspoon salt.

4 For dressing, whisk remaining ¼ cup olive oil, ¼ teaspoon cumin and lime juice in medium bowl. Season with salt and pepper.

5 Arrange lettuce on large serving platter. Top with quinoa mixture, tomatoes, avocado, cheese, tortilla strips and pepitas. Serve with dressing.

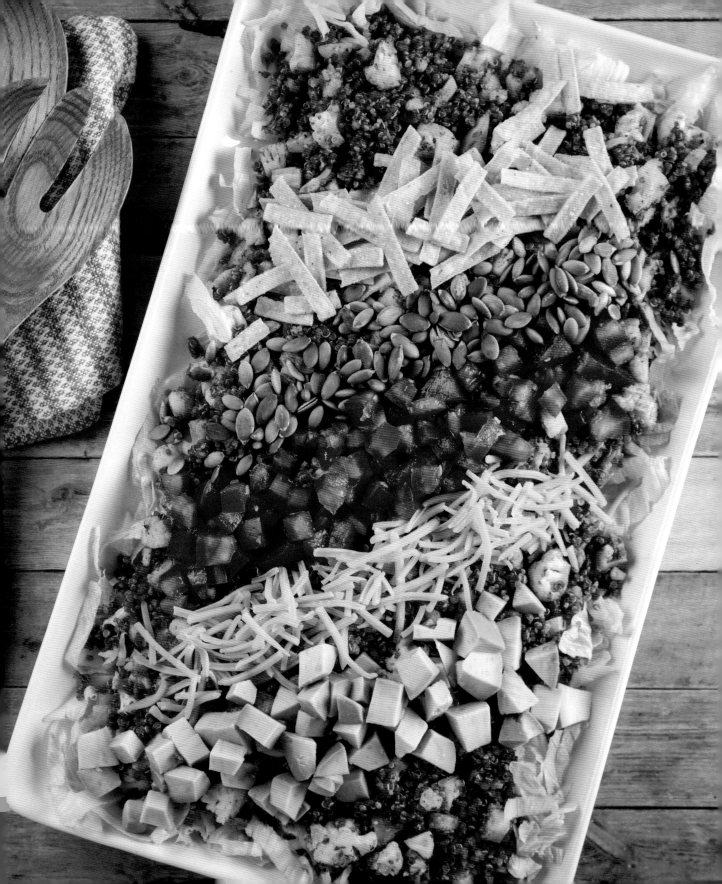

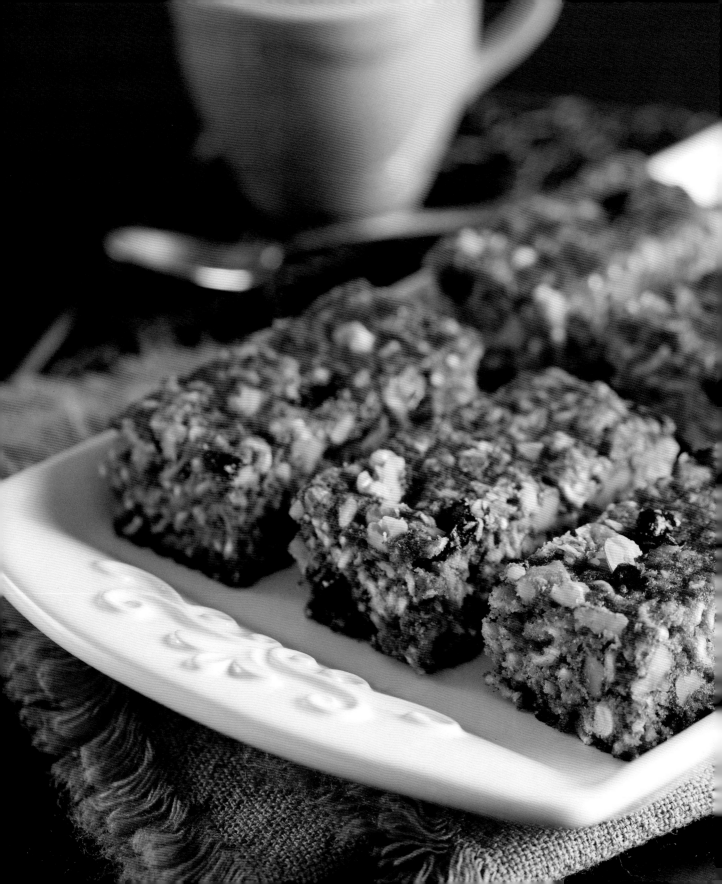

SWEET ENDINGS

CRANBERRY WALNUT GRANOLA BARS

2 cups old-fashioned oats

¾ cup all-purpose flour

1 teaspoon pumpkin pie spice

½ teaspoon baking soda

½ teaspoon salt

1 cup packed brown sugar

¼ cup (½ stick) butter, softened

2 eggs

¼ cup orange juice

1 cup chopped walnuts

½ cup dried cranberries

1 Preheat oven to 350°F. Spray 9-inch square baking pan with nonstick cooking spray.

2 Combine oats, flour, pumpkin pie spice, baking soda and salt in medium bowl.

3 Beat brown sugar and butter in large bowl with electric mixer at medium-high speed until light and fluffy. Add eggs and orange juice; beat until blended. Gradually add oat mixture, beating just until mixed. Stir in walnuts and cranberries. Spread mixture in prepared pan.

4 Bake 20 to 25 minutes or until toothpick inserted into center comes out clean. Cool completely in pan. Cut into bars.

CHAI SPICED BROWN RICE & CHIA PUDDING

MAKES 4 SERVINGS

4 English breakfast tea bags

4 cups plain unsweetened soymilk or almond milk

½ cup uncooked short grain brown rice, rinsed well

¼ cup chia seeds

2 tablespoons packed brown sugar

2 tablespoons agave nectar

1 teaspoon ground cinnamon

½ teaspoon ground ginger

¼ teaspoon salt

¼ teaspoon ground cardamom

¼ cup raisins

Whipped topping (optional)

1 Pour 1 cup boiling water over tea bags in liquid measuring cup. Steep 5 minutes; discard tea bags.

2 Combine tea, soymilk, rice, chia seeds, brown sugar, agave, cinnamon, ginger, salt and cardamom in large saucepan. Bring to a boil over medium-high heat. Reduce heat to low.

3 Cook, partially covered, 1½ hours or until rice is tender and mixture is thick and creamy, stirring occasionally. Skim off any film that appears on surface. Stir in raisins.

4 Serve warm or at room temperature. Top with whipped topping, if desired.

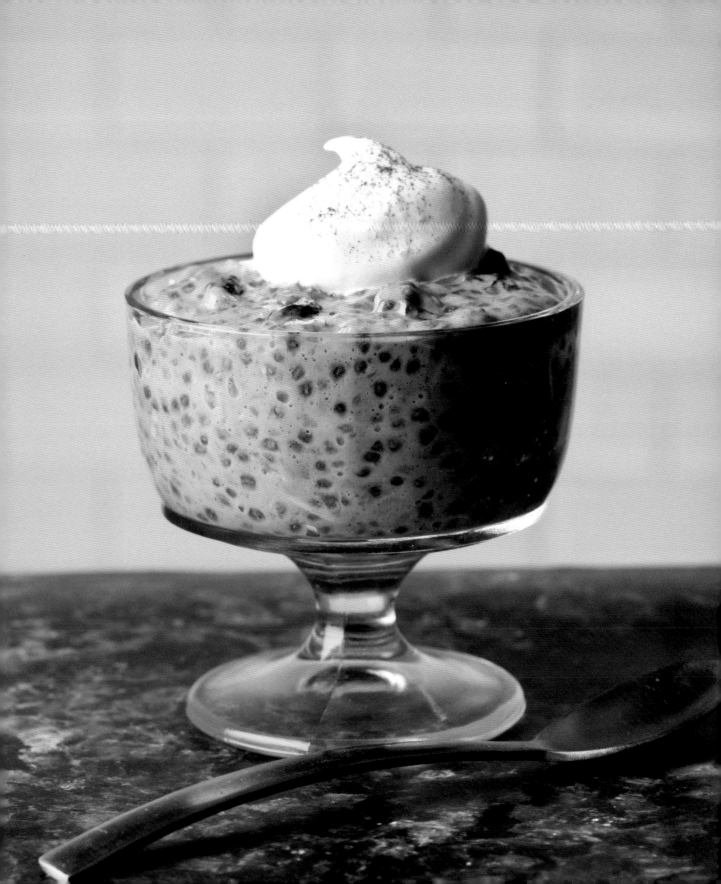

BANANA OATMEAL COOKIES

MAKES ABOUT 3 DOZEN COOKIES

⅓ cup plus 6 tablespoons boiling water, divided

2 tablespoons ground flaxseed

1 cup raisins

2 cups old-fashioned oats

2 cups all-purpose flour

1 tablespoon ground cinnamon

1 teaspoon baking soda

1 teaspoon salt

½ teaspoon ground nutmeg

¼ teaspoon ground cardamom

1½ cups sugar

¾ cup (1½ sticks) butter, softened

2 eggs

3 bananas, mashed

½ cup chopped pecans

1 Preheat oven to 375°F. Stir 6 tablespoons boiling water into flaxseed in small bowl. Cool completely; refrigerate until ready to use. Place raisins in small bowl. Pour remaining ⅓ cup boiling water over raisins; set aside.

2 Combine oats, flour, cinnamon, baking soda, salt, nutmeg and cardamom in medium bowl. Beat sugar and butter in large bowl with electric mixer at medium speed until creamy. Add eggs, bananas and flaxseed mixture; beat until well blended. Gradually add oat mixture; beat at low speed until stiff dough forms. Drain raisins. Stir in raisins and pecans. Drop dough by heaping tablespoonfuls 2 inches apart onto ungreased cookie sheets.

3 Bake 10 to 12 minutes or until edges are set and lightly browned. Cool on cookie sheets 1 minute. Remove to wire racks; cool completely.

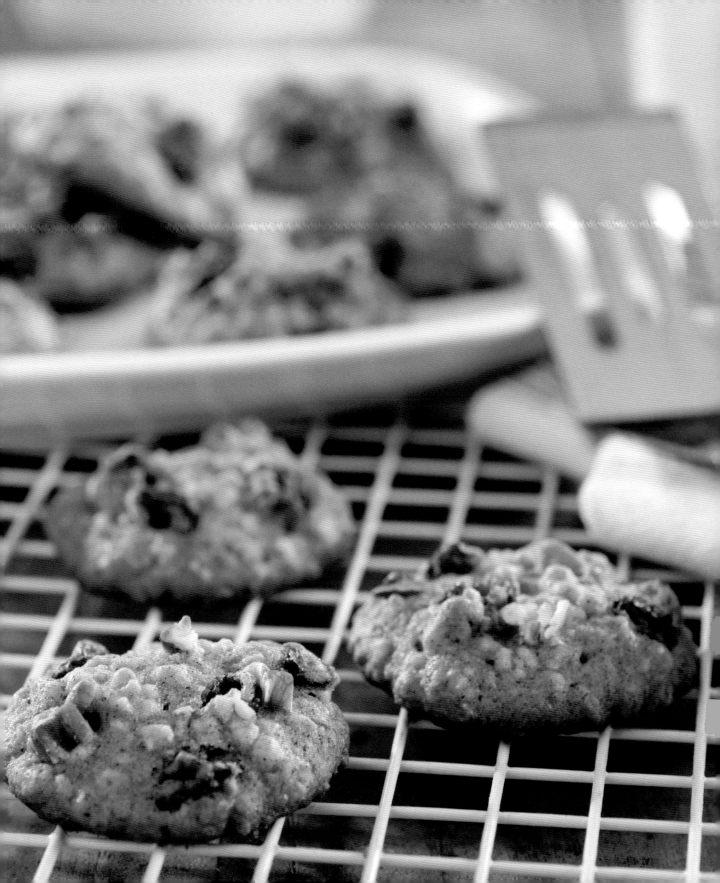

VEGAN CHOCOLATE CAKE

MAKES 12 TO 16 SERVINGS

Cake

- 6 tablespoons boiling water
- 2 tablespoons ground flaxseed
- 2 cups granulated sugar
- 2 cups all-purpose flour
- 1 cup unsweetened cocoa powder
- 1 tablespoon instant espresso powder*
- 2 teaspoons baking soda
- 1½ teaspoons baking powder
- 1½ teaspoons salt
- ¾ cup plain unsweetened almond milk
- ½ cup vegetable oil
- 1 tablespoon apple cider vinegar
- 2 teaspoons vanilla
- 1 cup hot water*

Frosting

- 1 package (12 ounces) vegan chocolate chips
- ¼ teaspoon salt
- 1 can (about 13 ounces) full-fat coconut milk
- 2 cups powdered sugar

Or substitute 1 cup hot strong brewed coffee.

1 Preheat oven to 350°F. Line 13×9-inch baking pan with parchment paper or spray with nonstick cooking spray. Combine boiling water and flaxseed in small bowl; cool completely.

2 Whisk granulated sugar, flour, cocoa, espresso powder, baking soda, baking powder and 1½ teaspoons salt in large bowl. Make well in center. Pour almond milk, oil, vinegar, vanilla and flaxseed mixture into well; whisk gently to blend wet ingredients. Whisk into dry ingredients until moistened. Add hot water; whisk until well blended. Pour into prepared pan.

3 Bake 35 to 40 minutes or until top appears dry and toothpick inserted into center comes out clean. Cool completely in pan on wire rack.

4 For frosting, place chocolate chips and ¼ teaspoon salt in bowl of electric stand mixer. Bring coconut milk to a simmer in small saucepan over medium heat, whisking frequently to blend. Pour 1 cup coconut milk over chips; swirl to coat. Let stand 5 minutes; whisk until smooth. Cool to room temperature.** Add powdered sugar; beat at low speed until blended. Increase speed to medium-high; beat 1 to 2 minutes or until frosting is fluffy and smooth. If frosting is too thick, add remaining coconut milk by teaspoonfuls until desired consistency is reached.

**To frost cake with ganache instead of frosting, spread cooled mixture over top of cake (skip the powdered sugar). For firm ganache, refrigerate until set.

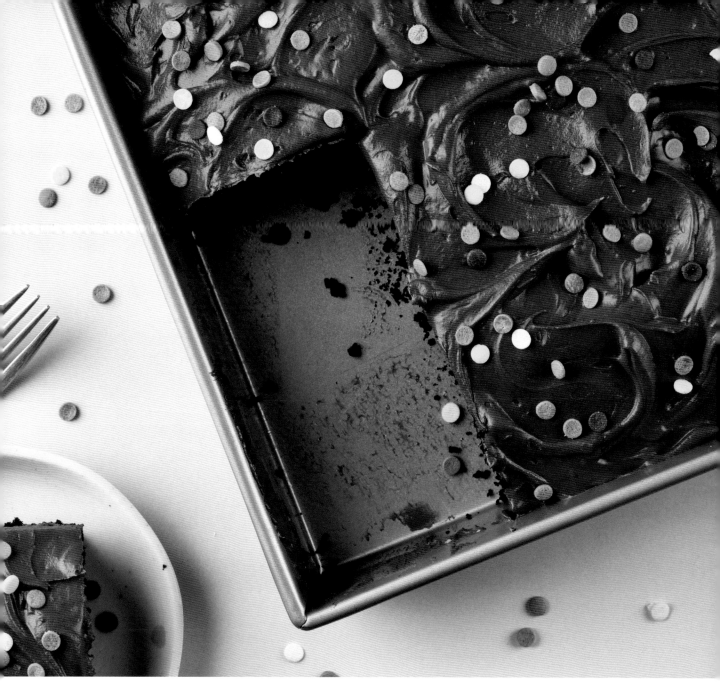

Note

This cake keeps very well at room temperature (frosted or unfrosted) for a few days—just cover it tightly with plastic wrap. To make the neatest slices, run a long sharp knife (not serrated) under hot water to warm it and wipe dry immediately. After every cut, rewarm it under hot water and wipe dry as needed.

WHOLE GRAIN CRANBERRY CHOCOLATE CHIP COOKIES

MAKES ABOUT 18 COOKIES

1½ cups five-grain cereal, uncooked

1 cup whole wheat flour

½ teaspoon salt

½ teaspoon baking soda

¼ teaspoon baking powder

½ cup (1 stick) unsalted butter, softened

⅓ cup packed brown sugar

1 egg

½ teaspoon vanilla

½ cup golden raisins

½ cup semisweet chocolate chips

½ cup sweetened dried cranberries, chopped

1 Preheat oven to 350°F. Spray nonstick cookie sheet with nonstick cooking spray. Combine cereal, flour, salt, baking soda and baking powder in medium bowl.

2 Beat butter and brown sugar in large bowl with electric mixer at medium speed until light and fluffy. Beat in egg and vanilla until well blended. Beat in flour mixture just until blended. Fold in raisins, chocolate chips and cranberries. Drop dough by tablespoonfuls 2 inches apart onto prepared cookie sheet.

3 Bake in center of oven 7 to 9 minutes or until golden. Transfer cookies to wire rack to cool completely.

Variations

Substitute other multigrain cooked cereals for the five-grain cereal. For additional flavor variations, you can also experiment with other dried fruit, such as dried apricots or cherries. Just be sure to chop the fruit well to evenly distribute it among the cookies.

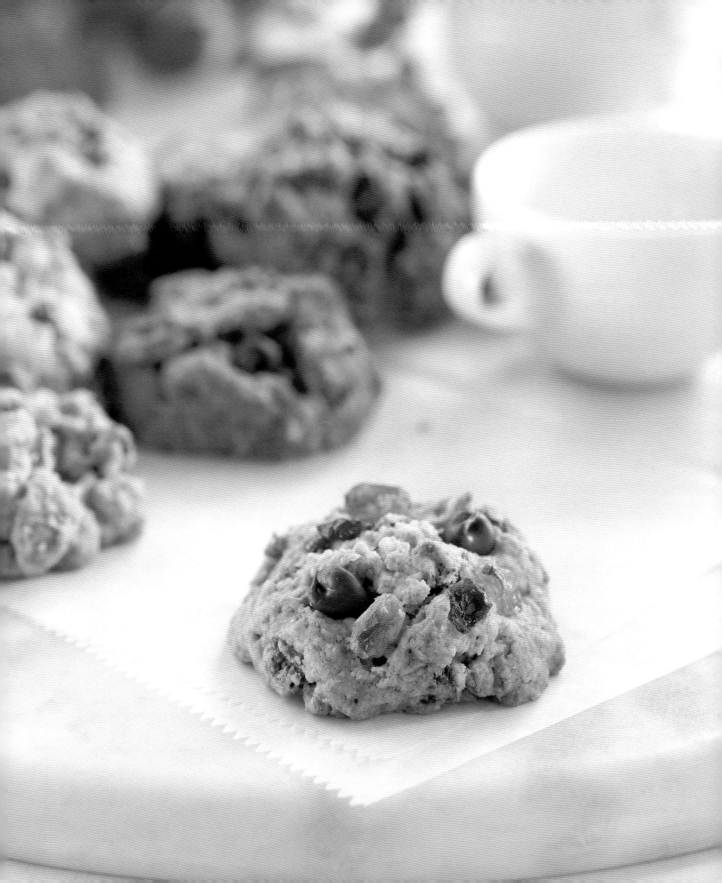

MIXED BERRY WHOLE GRAIN COFFEECAKE

MAKES 12 SERVINGS

1¼ cups all-purpose flour, divided

¾ cup quick oats

¾ cup packed light brown sugar

3 tablespoons butter, softened

1 cup whole wheat flour

1 cup fat-free (skim) milk

¾ cup granulated sugar

¼ cup canola oil

1 egg, slightly beaten

1 tablespoon baking powder

1 teaspoon ground cinnamon

½ teaspoon salt

1½ cups frozen unsweetened mixed berries, thawed and drained *or* 2 cups fresh berries

¼ cup chopped walnuts

1 Preheat oven to 350°F. Spray 9×5-inch loaf pan with nonstick cooking spray.

2 Combine ¼ cup all-purpose flour, oats, brown sugar and butter in small bowl; mix with fork until crumbly.

3 Combine remaining 1 cup all-purpose flour, whole wheat flour, milk, granulated sugar, oil, egg, baking powder, cinnamon and salt in large bowl. Beat with electric mixer or whisk 1 to 2 minutes until well blended. Fold in berries. Spread batter in prepared pan; sprinkle evenly with oat mixture and walnuts.

4 Bake 38 to 40 minutes or until toothpick inserted into center comes out clean. Serve warm.

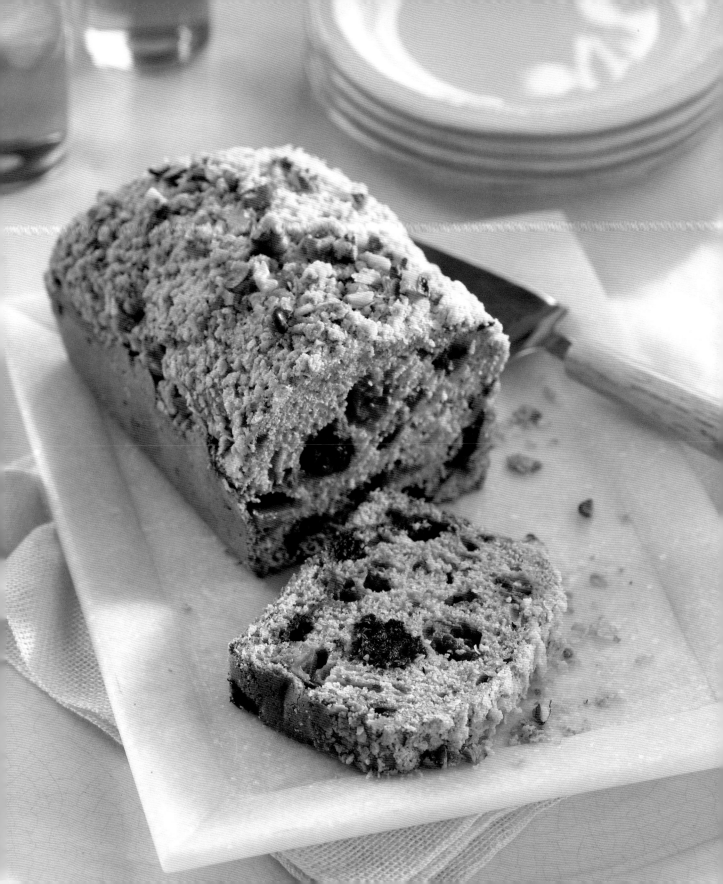

CINNAMON-WHEAT
BROWNIES

MAKES 16 BROWNIES

2 ounces unsweetened
   chocolate, chopped

½ cup (1 stick) butter,
   softened

1 cup packed dark brown
   sugar

2 eggs

1 teaspoon ground cinnamon

1 teaspoon vanilla

¼ teaspoon baking powder

¼ teaspoon ground ginger

⅛ teaspoon ground cloves

½ cup whole wheat flour

1 cup coarsely chopped
   walnuts

1 Preheat oven to 350°F. Butter 8-inch square baking
  pan. Melt chocolate in top of double boiler over
  simmering water. Cool.

2 Beat butter, sugar, eggs and melted chocolate in large
  bowl with electric mixer at medium speed until light
  and smooth. Blend in cinnamon, vanilla, baking
  powder, ginger and cloves. Stir in flour and walnuts
  until well blended. Spread batter evenly in prepared
  pan.

3 Bake 25 minutes or until top feels firm and dry. Cool
  completely in pan on wire rack. Cut into 2-inch
  squares.

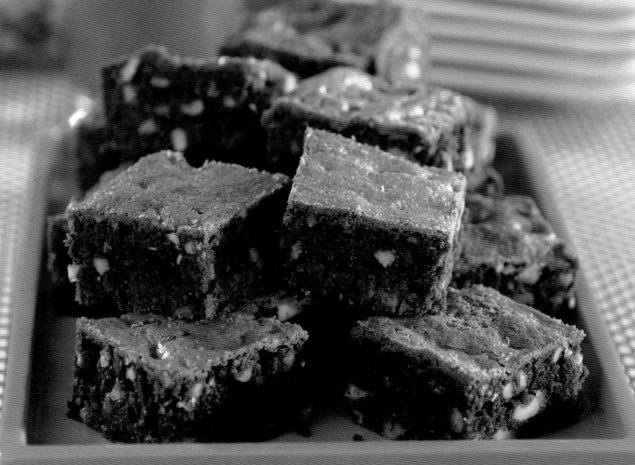

NO-BAKE FRUIT AND GRAIN BARS

MAKES 16 BARS

½ cup cooked amaranth*

2 cups whole grain puffed rice cereal

½ cup chopped dried fruit

½ cup honey

¼ cup sugar

¾ cup almond butter

*Amaranth can be found in health food stores in the bulk bins. It may also be found in large supermarkets in the health food aisle.

1 Spray 8- or 9-inch square baking pan with nonstick cooking spray.

2 Heat medium saucepan over high heat. Add 1 tablespoon amaranth; stir or gently shake saucepan until almost all seeds have popped. (Partially cover saucepan if seeds are popping over the side.) Remove to medium bowl. Repeat with remaining amaranth.

3 Stir cereal and dried fruit into popped amaranth.

4 Combine honey and sugar in same saucepan; bring to a boil over medium heat. Remove from heat; stir in almond butter until melted and smooth.

5 Pour honey mixture over cereal mixture; stir until evenly coated. Press firmly into prepared pan. Let stand until set. Cut into bars.

Note

Amaranth is a gluten-free whole grain that's high in protein and fiber. Cooked amaranth is tender with a slight crunch. It doesn't fluff up like rice, but instead has a dense quality that retains moisture.

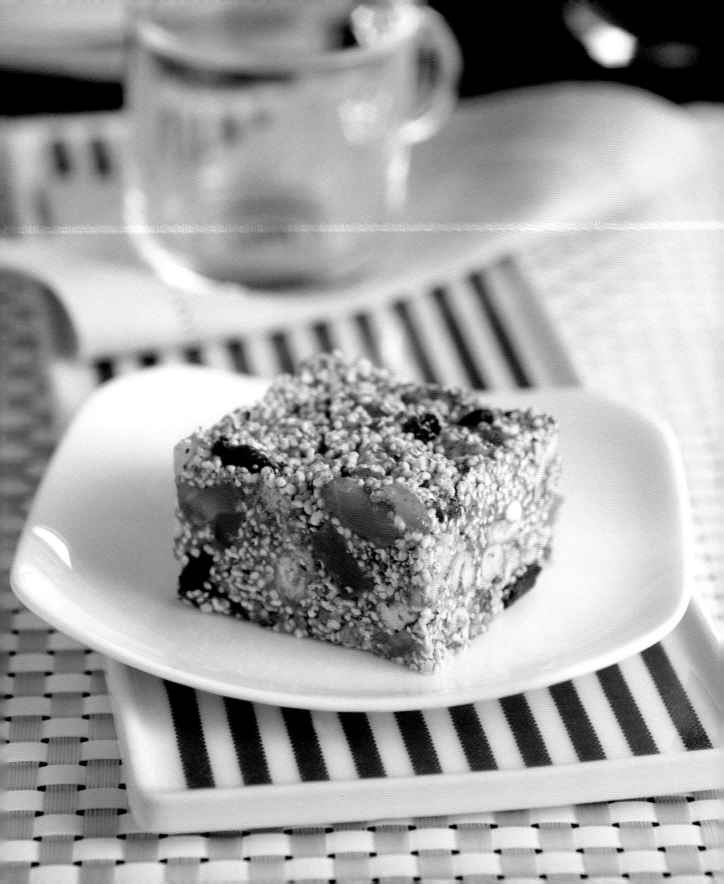

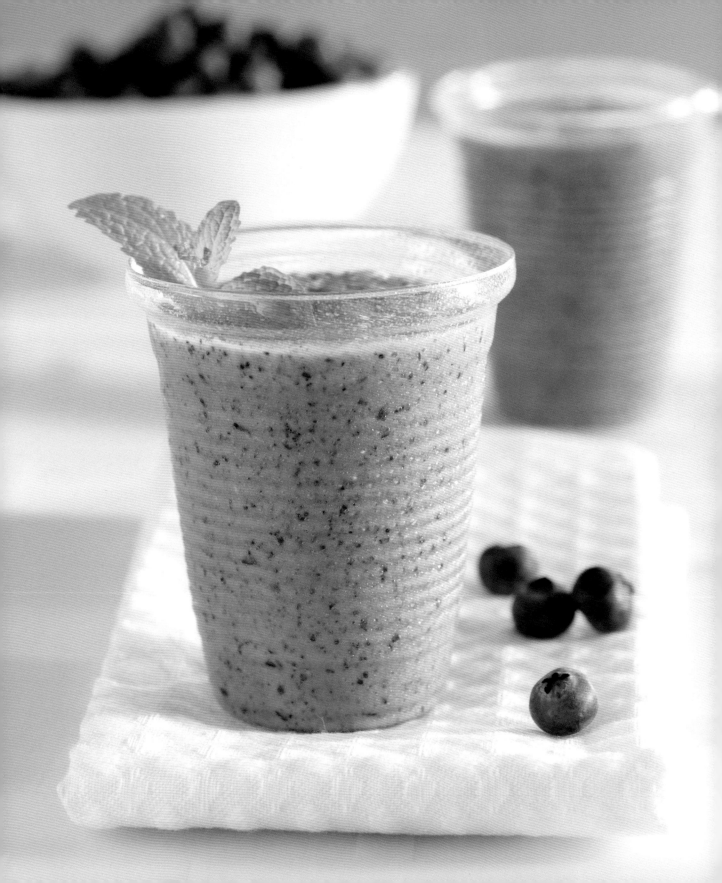

SMOOTHIES & JUICES

BLUEBERRY BANANA OATMEAL SMOOTHIE

MAKES 2 SERVINGS

1 cup oat milk

1 small ripe banana

½ cup frozen blueberries

1 container (5 ounces) nondairy yogurt (about ½ cup)

¼ cup quick oats

1 Combine milk, banana and blueberries in blender; blend until smooth. Add yogurt and oats; blend until smooth.

2 Pour into 2 glasses.

CRANBERRY PEAR GINGER SMOOTHIE

MAKES 2 SERVINGS

2 cups peeled diced pears *or* 1 can (15 ounces) sliced pears, drained

1½ cups apple juice

½ cup whole berry cranberry sauce

½ teaspoon ground ginger

2 to 3 ice cubes

1 Combine pears and apple juice in blender; blend until smooth. Add cranberry sauce and ginger; blend until smooth. Add ice; blend until smooth.

2 Pour into 2 glasses.

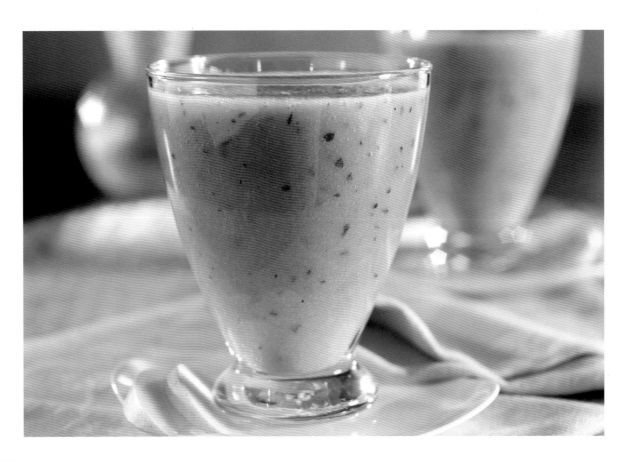

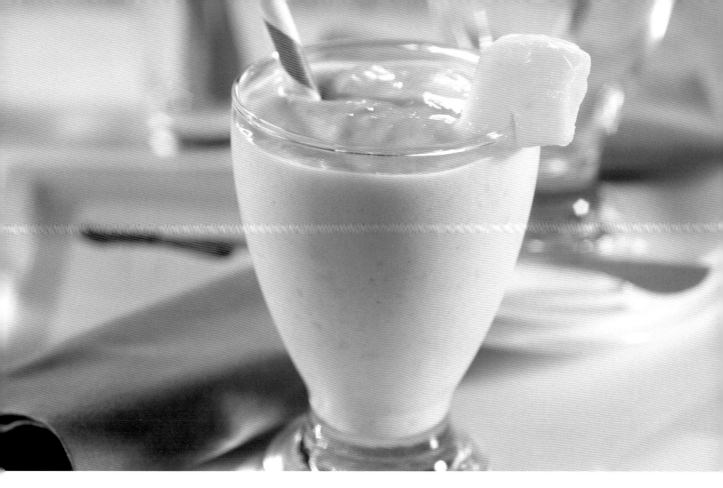

MANGO SMOOTHIE

2 cups frozen mango chunks, plus additional for garnish

2 containers (6 ounces each) vanilla low-fat yogurt

¾ cup orange juice

1 teaspoon vanilla (optional)

Juice of ½ lime

Pinch salt

1 Combine 2 cups mango chunks, yogurt, orange juice, vanilla, if desired, lime juice and salt in blender; blend until smooth.

2 Pour into 4 glasses. Garnish with additional mango chunks.

Note

If you can't find frozen mango chunks, you can make your own. Cut mango into 1-inch chunks; place on cookie sheet and freeze for about 3 hours.

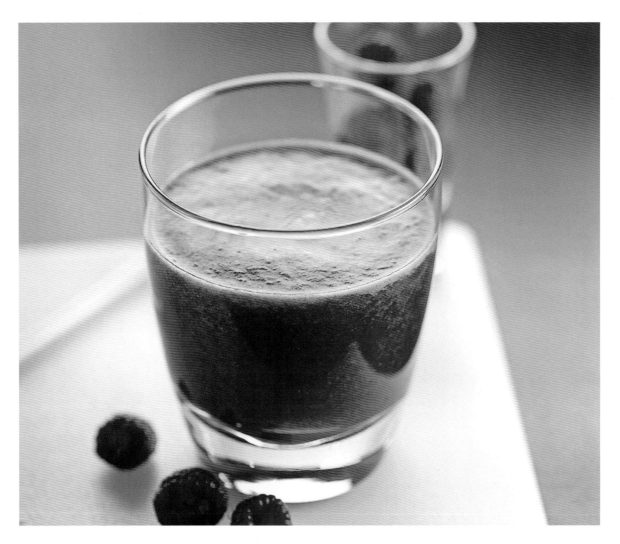

ORCHARD
CRUSH

MAKES 2 SERVINGS

2 apples
1 cup fresh raspberries
1 cup fresh strawberries

Juice apples, raspberries and strawberries. Stir.

APPLE-K
JUICE

MAKES 2 SERVINGS

1 kiwi, peeled

1 apple

4 leaves kale

1 stalk celery

½ lemon, peeled

Juice kiwi, apple, kale, celery and lemon. Stir.

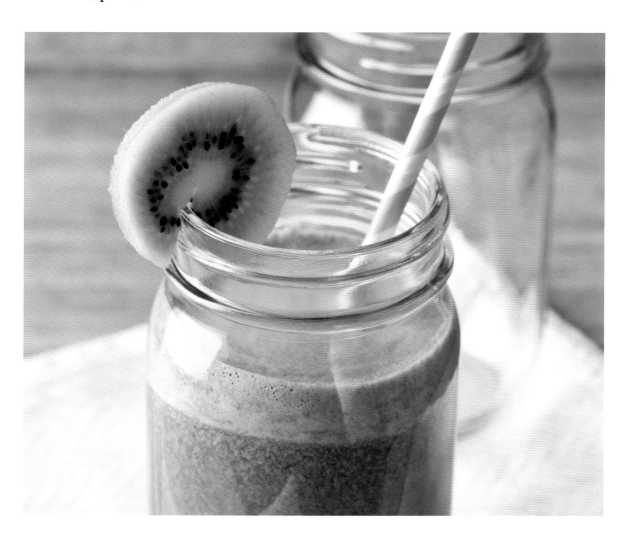

PURPLEBERRY JUICE

MAKES 2 SERVINGS

2 cups red seedless grapes

1 apple

½ cup fresh blackberries

½ inch fresh ginger, peeled

Juice grapes, apple, blackberries and ginger. Stir.

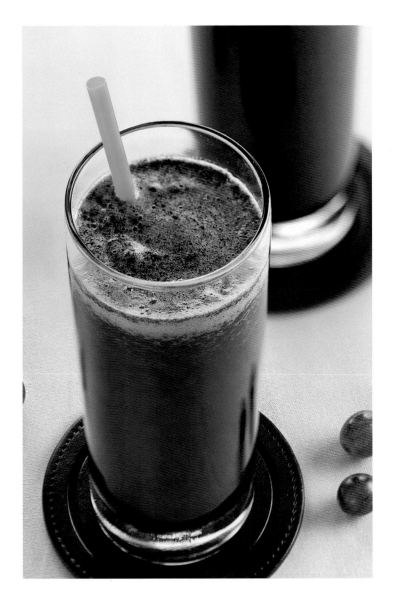

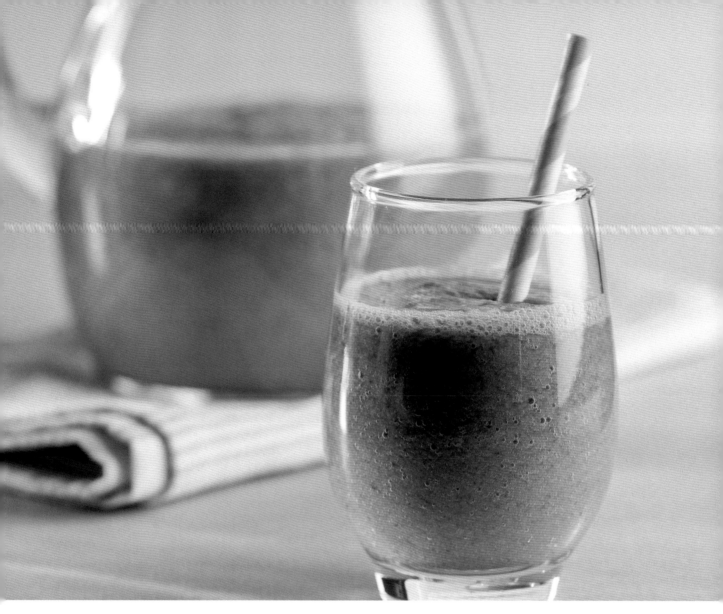

TANGY APPLE
KALE SMOOTHIE

MAKES 3 SERVINGS

1 cup water

2 Granny Smith apples, seeded and cut into chunks

2 cups baby kale

1 frozen banana

Combine water, apples, kale and banana in blender; blend until smooth. Serve immediately.

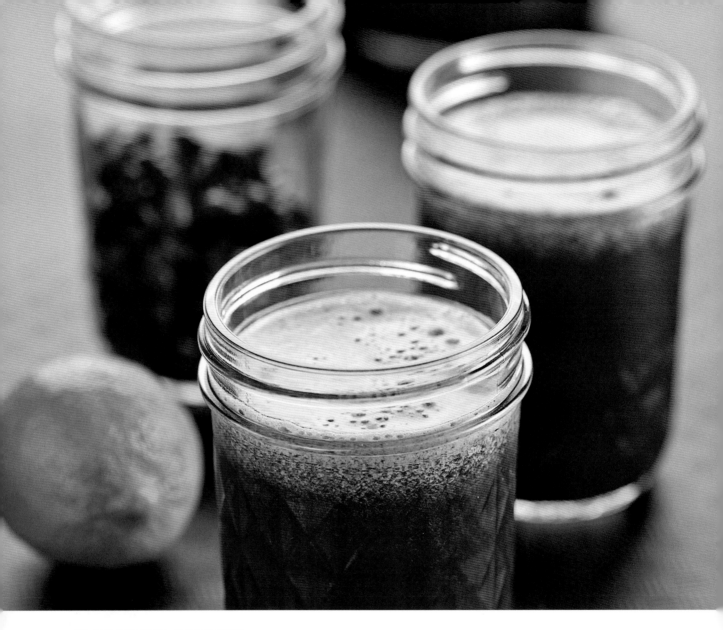

POMEGRANATE-LIME-COCONUT JUICE

1 pomegranate, peeled

½ cucumber

1 lime, peeled

¼ cup coconut water

Juice pomegranate seeds, cucumber and lime. Stir in coconut water until well blended.

CUCUMBER
BASIL COOLER

1 cucumber

1 apple

½ cup fresh basil

½ lime, peeled

Juice cucumber, apple, basil and lime. Stir.

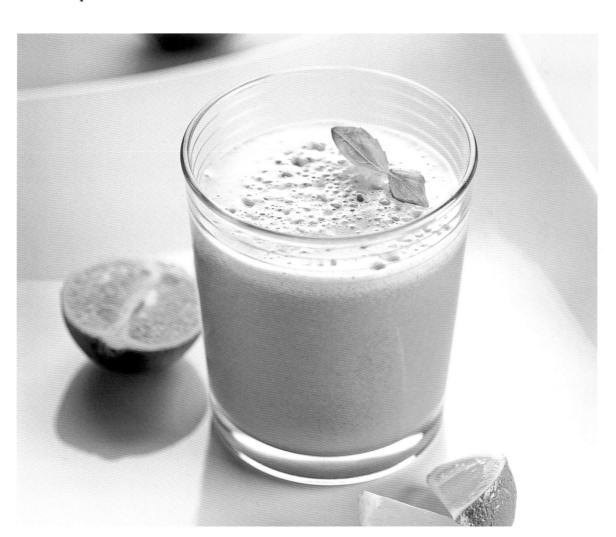

CLEANSING GREEN JUICE

MAKES 2 SERVINGS

4 leaves bok choy

1 stalk celery

½ cucumber

¼ bulb fennel

½ lemon, peeled

Juice bok choy, celery, cucumber, fennel and lemon. Stir.

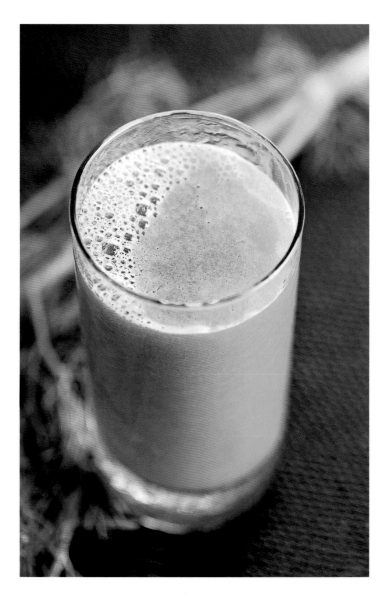

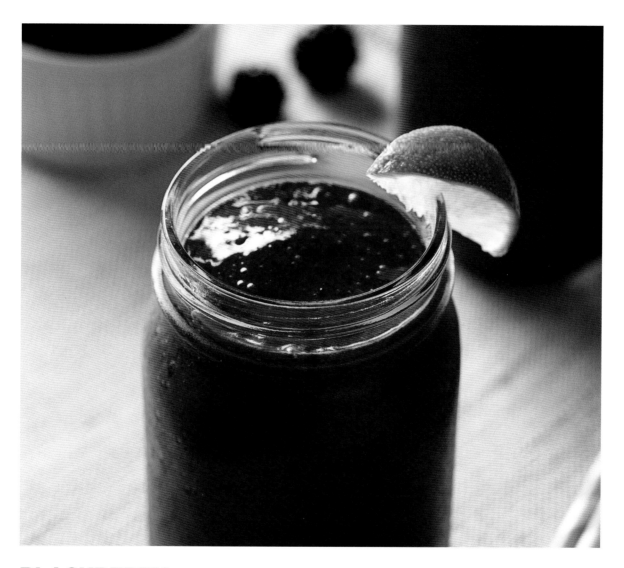

BLACKBERRY
LIME SMOOTHIE

MAKES 1 SERVING

1 cup frozen blackberries

1 cup reduced-fat (2%) milk

1 tablespoon sugar

1 tablespoon fresh lime juice

Combine blackberries, milk, sugar and lime juice in blender; blend until smooth.

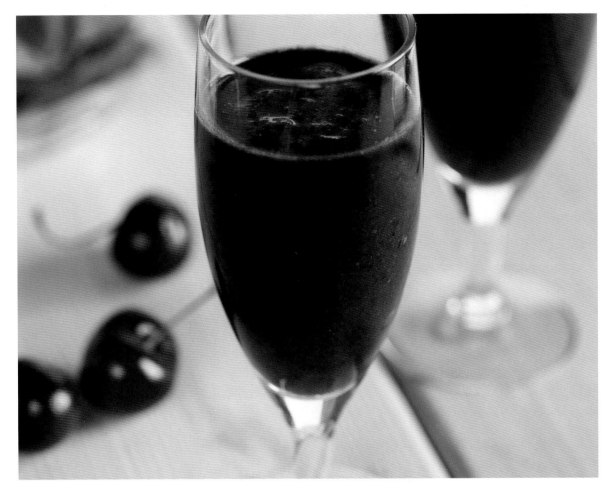

CHERRY GREEN SMOOTHIE

MAKES 2 SERVINGS

¾ cup almond milk

1½ cups frozen dark sweet cherries

¾ cup baby spinach

½ frozen banana

1 tablespoon ground flaxseed

2 teaspoons honey (optional)

Combine almond milk, cherries, spinach, banana, flaxseed and honey, if desired, in blender; blend until smooth. Serve immediately.

SALAD BAR SMOOTHIE

1½ cups ice cubes

½ banana

½ cup fresh raspberries

½ cup sliced fresh strawberries

½ cup fresh blueberries

½ cup packed torn spinach

Combine ice, banana, raspberries, strawberries, blueberries and spinach in blender; blend until smooth.

Note

Fresh or frozen berries can be used to make this recipe. When using frozen fruit, reduce the amount of ice used.

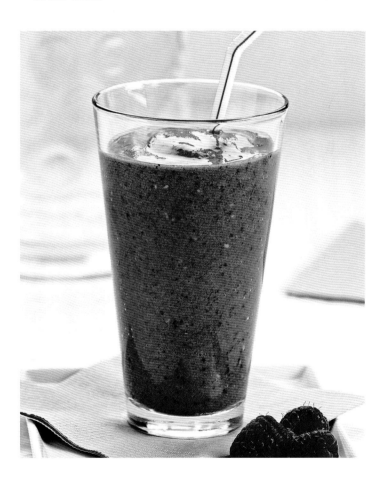

JOINT
COMFORT
JUICE

MAKES 2 SERVINGS

2 cups fresh spinach

¼ pineapple, peeled

1 pear

1 cup fresh parsley

½ grapefruit, peeled

Juice spinach, pineapple, pear, parsley and grapefruit. Stir.

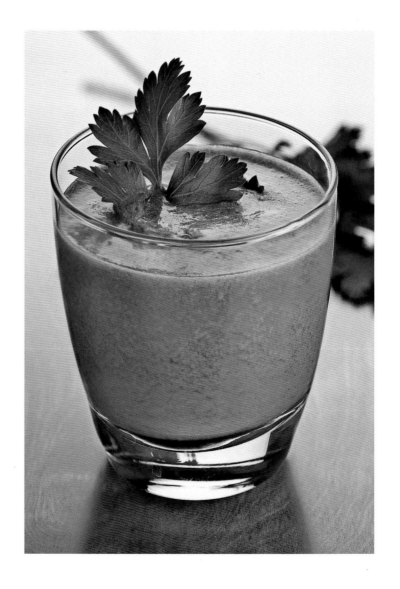

METRIC CONVERSION CHART

VOLUME MEASUREMENTS (dry)

⅛ teaspoon = 0.5 mL
¼ teaspoon = 1 mL
½ teaspoon = 2 mL
¾ teaspoon = 4 mL
1 teaspoon = 5 mL
1 tablespoon = 15 mL
2 tablespoons = 30 mL
¼ cup = 60 mL
⅓ cup = 75 mL
½ cup = 125 mL
⅔ cup = 150 mL
¾ cup = 175 mL
1 cup = 250 mL
2 cups = 1 pint = 500 mL
3 cups = 750 mL
4 cups = 1 quart = 1 L

VOLUME MEASUREMENTS (fluid)

1 fluid ounce (2 tablespoons) = 30 mL
4 fluid ounces (½ cup) = 125 mL
8 fluid ounces (1 cup) = 250 mL
12 fluid ounces (1½ cups) = 375 mL
16 fluid ounces (2 cups) = 500 mL

WEIGHTS (mass)

½ ounce = 15 g
1 ounce = 30 g
3 ounces = 90 g
4 ounces = 120 g
8 ounces = 225 g
10 ounces = 285 g
12 ounces = 360 g
16 ounces = 1 pound = 450 g

DIMENSIONS

1/16 inch = 2 mm
⅛ inch = 3 mm
¼ inch = 6 mm
½ inch = 1.5 cm
¾ inch = 2 cm
1 inch = 2.5 cm

OVEN TEMPERATURES

250°F = 120°C
275°F = 140°C
300°F = 150°C
325°F = 160°C
350°F = 180°C
375°F = 190°C
400°F = 200°C
425°F = 220°C
450°F = 230°C

BAKING PAN SIZES

Utensil	Size in Inches/Quarts	Metric Volume	Size in Centimeters
Baking or Cake Pan (square or rectangular)	8×8×2	2 L	20×20×5
	9×9×2	2.5 L	23×23×5
	12×8×2	3 L	30×20×5
	13×9×2	3.5 L	33×23×5
Loaf Pan	8×4×3	1.5 L	20×10×7
	9×5×3	2 L	23×13×7
Round Layer Cake Pan	8×1½	1.2 L	20×4
	9×1½	1.5 L	23×4
Pie Plate	8×1¼	750 mL	20×3
	9×1¼	1 L	23×3
Baking Dish or Casserole	1 quart	1 L	—
	1½ quart	1.5 L	—
	2 quart	2 L	—